MANAGEMENT

OF

HYPERTENSION

by

Norman M. Kaplan, M.D.

Department of Internal Medicine
University of Texas
Southwestern Medical School
5323 Harry Hines Boulevard
Dallas, Texas 75235-8899

Fourth Edition

**Essential Medical
Information Systems, Inc.**
Durant, OK

Direct Mail Orders
Essential Medical
Information Systems, Inc.
P.O. Box 1607
Durant, OK 74702-1607

Telephone Orders

1-800-225-0694
FAX Your Order: (405) 924-9414

FOURTH EDITION

ISBN: 0-929240-34-0

Published in the United States 1992

Center Index Texts Published By
Essential Medical Information Systems, Inc.

TABLE OF CONTENTS

TABLES

FIGURES

Foreword

This book, hopefully, will prove useful to those who want a ready up-to-date reference to practical issues in the treatment of hypertensive patients. My larger book, *Clinical Hypertension*, now in its 5th edition, should provide additional background, detail and references for those who need them.

I thank all of my co-workers, both in Dallas and elsewhere, who have provided me with the data and the insights needed to write this book.

#1 Measurement of Blood Pressure

General Principles

The first and most important step in the management of hypertension is a careful assessment of the level of the blood pressure. It must be taken frequently and carefully. The blood pressure naturally varies a great deal so it is important to avoid all controllable causes of variation. During 24 hour ambulatory monitoring, pressures while awake may vary by more than 30 mm Hg, with highest levels usually noted in the early morning and lower readings in the afternoon. Much lower levels are usual during sleep, with the important exception of higher readings during periods of sleep apnea.

Establishing the Diagnosis

At least three sets of three readings should be taken with intervals of two weeks or more between each set unless the initial level is so high (above 180/110) or target organ damage is so ominous as to demand immediate intervention. Even more readings may be obtained, preferably at various times and under various circumstances with inexpensive, semiautomatic, home devices.

Levels of blood pressure tend to fall after the first reading with most of the fall noted during the first few weeks. Most home readings are 5 to 10 mm Hg lower than those obtained in the office.

Even though the initial higher office readings may indicate higher risks for the subsequent development of cardiovascular disease, the average of multiple readings taken over one to two months should be taken to establish the diagnosis of hypertension and to decide upon the need for therapy.

Monitoring Progress

For many, only occasional follow-up readings are needed, initially more frequently than later. If changes in therapy are made, readings should be taken after two to four weeks unless side effects occur. Once the goal of therapy is reached and the patient is asymptomatic, readings need only be obtained every four to six months.

For others, more frequent readings taken out of the office will be useful. These include patients with:

- Poor control based on office blood pressure despite increasing medication
- Advancing target organ damage despite apparent good control based on office readings
- Symptoms that could reflect hypotension

In addition, home readings are needed to ensure 24 hour control of hypertension with a particular need to document that the early morning surge in pressure is moderated in hopes of avoiding the high incidence of cardiovascular catastrophes between 6:00 and 10:00 a.m.

Basic Technique

The basic technique in the measurement of the blood pressure includes:

- At least two readings at each visit; if they differ by more than 5 mm Hg, additional readings should be taken
- On initial visit supine and standing readings may be indicated, particularly in elderly and diabetics
- Measure blood pressure in both arms; if there is a persistent difference, use arm with higher pressure
- The patient should sit in a chair for at least five minutes with the arm unconstricted and supported at the level of the heart on a platform or table
- Avoid extraneous factors which may alter pressure or, if unavoidable, make note of:
  - Smoking or eating within the prior 30 minutes
  - Anxiety
  - Talking
  - Exertion
  - Cold
  - Bladder distention

- Medications, which include:
  - Estrogens
  - Adrenal steroids
  - Adrenergic drugs such as nose drops or 10 percent phenylephrine used to dilate pupils for funduscopic exam
- Note the time of day
- Use proper sized cuff, ie, the largest that will fit the upper arm is appropriate
- Inflate bladder to above systolic level by palpating the disappearance of the radial pulse. If radial artery remains palpable after pulse disappears, consider "pseudo-hypertension" from calcified vessels which cannot be collapsed beneath bladder
- Deflate cuff at rate of 2 to 3 mm Hg per heart beat
- Use disappearance of sound (Korotkoff V) as diastolic level
- In patients below age 20 or if femoral pulse is weak, take pressure in one leg

(From Kaplan, NM: *Clinical Hypertension, 5th ed.*, 1990.)

References

1989 Guidelines for the management of mild hypertension: Memorandum from a WHO/ISH meeting. Hypertension 1989; 7:689-693.

Evans CE, et al: Home blood pressure-measuring devices: A comparative study of accuracy. J Hypertension 1989;7:133-142.

Kaplan NM: Misdiagnosis of systemic hypertension and recommendations for improvement (Editorial). Am J Cardiol 1987; 60:1383-1386.

Mancia G, et al: Alerting reaction and rise in blood pressure during measurement by physician and nurse. Hypertension 1987;9:209-215.

Muller JE, Tofler GH: A symposium: Triggering and circadian variation of onset of acute cardiovascular disease. Am J Cardiol 1990;66:1G-70G.

O'Brien E, Fitzgerald D, O'Malley K: Blood pressure measurement: Current practice and future trends. Br Med J 1985; 290:729-734.

Perloff D, Sokolow M, Cowan R: The prognostic value of ambulatory blood pressure. JAMA 1983;249:2792-2798.

Pickering TG, et al: How common is white coat hypertension? JAMA 1988;259:225-228.

Siegel WC, Blumenthal JA, Divine GW: Physiological, psychological, and behavioral factors and white coat hypertension. Hypertension 1990;16:140-146.

Weber MA: Whole-day blood pressure. Hypertension 1988; 11:288-298.

#2 Definition of Hypertension

General Definition

The long-term risks for the development of cardio-vascular disease increase with every increment of blood pressure. The degree of risk for coronary and cerebral vascular disease is some two-fold higher in adults with diastolic blood pressure (DBP) above 90 mm Hg compared to those with DBP below 80. The definition of hypertension is usually based on DBP but the presence of isolated elevations of systolic blood pressure (SBP) above 160 mm Hg, usually seen in people over age 65, is associated with a significantly higher risk, particularly for stroke.

Based on the relative increase in risks, hypertension may be defined as sustained average levels of blood pressure above 140/90 mm Hg in adult patients. Those with DBP below 90 but SBP above 160 may be defined as having isolated systolic hypertension. These levels have been proposed as the upper limit of normal for children:

Age/Years	Blood Pressure
13 to 15	136/86
10 to 12	126/82
6 to 9	122/78
3 to 5	116/76

Classification by Degree

The 1988 Joint National Committee report proposed this classification of the degree of hypertension:

Range of Blood Pressure	Category of Hypertension
Diastolic	
90 to 104	Mild hypertension
105 to 114	Moderate hypertension
115 and above	Severe hypertension
Systolic (DBP < 90)	
140 to 159	Borderline isolated systolic hypertension
160 and above	Isolated systolic hypertension

The relative frequency of various categories of diastolic hypertension in a large population of people screened at home by the Hypertension Detection and Follow-up Program was about 80 percent mild, 15 percent moderate and 5 percent severe (Figure 2.1).

Those patients with DBP from 85 to 89 mm Hg may be classified as "high-normal." They should be more frequently rechecked and counseled more vigorously to follow the non-drug modalities (see Sections #9 and #10) which may decrease the likelihood for the progression of hypertension. Even if they do not, they should improve overall cardiovascular status at no financial cost and little interference with current life-style. Cessation of smoking, although it will not lower blood pressure, is the single most beneficial move to improve cardiovascular health.

Operational Definition

More than the risks of various levels of blood pressure should be considered before labeling a person as hypertensive. Logically, the label should be affixed only if active therapy is indicated. People labeled as hypertensive may suffer from increased psychoneurotic and other complaints, resulting in an increase in absenteeism from work. In addition, the label may be responsible for added economic burdens, eg, higher life insurance premiums and loss of job opportunities.

There is, then, a need to balance the risks of not diagnosing and treating a level of blood pressure against the costs and risk of doing so. In addition to the costs of labeling, there are risks from all currently used antihypertensive drugs. On the basis of current knowledge, most authorities agree that drug therapy be given to those with average DBP above 95 mm Hg, although some advocate that the level should be as low as 90 and others as high as 100 or even 105 (see Section #11).

From an operational viewpoint, many who are at increased risk need not be diagnosed as "hypertensive." However, they should be more carefully monitored and more vigorously counseled to improve their unhealthy life-styles. The label should be affixed to all with DBP that remains above 95 and, logically, to elderly with SBP above 160. Those with DBP between 85 and 94 or SBP between 140 and 159 who have few other risk factors may be more appropriately called "border-line" or "high-normal."

FIGURE 2.1 – The Distribution of Levels of Diastolic Blood Pressure

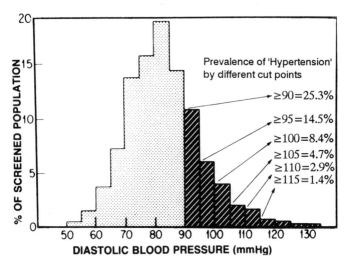

Frequency distribution of diastolic blood pressure at home screen (158,906 persons; 30 to 69 years of age). (From The Hypertension Detection and Follow-up Program. Circulation Research 40 (Supp I):106, 1977, by permission of the American Heart Association, Inc.)

References

Dannenberg AL, et al: Progress in the battle against hypertension. Changes in blood pressure levels in the United States from 1960 to 1980. Hypertension 1987;10:226-233.

Joint National Committee on Detection, Evaluation, and Treatment of High Blood Pressure: The 1988 report of the Joint National Committee on Detection, Evaluation, and Treatment of High Blood Pressure. Arch Intern Med 1988;148:1023-1038.

Julius S, et al: The association of borderline hypertension with target organ changes and higher coronary risk. Tecumseh Blood Pressure Study. JAMA 1990;264:354-358.

MacDonald LA, et al: Labeling in hypertension: A review of the behavioral and psychological consequences. J Chron Dis 1984;37:933-942.

MacMahon S, et al: Blood pressure, stroke, and coronary heart disease. Part 1, prolonged differences in blood pressure: Prospective observational studies corrected for the regression dilution bias. Lancet 1990;335:765-774.

Task Force on Blood Pressure Control in Children: Pediatrics. Report of the Second Task Force on Blood Pressure Control in Children-1987. Pediatrics 1987;79:11-24.

#3 Types of Hypertension

Primary Hypertension
Secondary Hypertension
Special Populations

3.

PRIMARY HYPERTENSION

In typical clinical practice, 95 percent of hypertensive adults aged 18 to 65 will have no identifiable cause, thus their hypertension should be defined either as primary or essential or idiopathic.

SECONDARY HYPERTENSION

The frequency of the secondary forms will likely approximate these figures:
- Renal parenchymal disease—3 to 4 percent
- Renal vascular hypertension—0.5 to 1 percent
- Adrenal hyperfunction—0.1 to 0.3 percent
  - Pheochromocytoma
  - Cushing's syndrome
  - Primary aldosteronism
- Miscellaneous causes—0.1 to 0.3 percent

SPECIAL POPULATIONS

Populations composed of varying proportions of special groups of patients will have different frequencies than those listed above.

Adults With Severe or Resistant Hypertension
Those with accelerated (Grade 3 fundi) or malignant (Grade 4 fundi) hypertension or whose hypertension remains resistant to appropriate therapy have a higher frequency of renal parenchymal disease and, even more so, of renal vascular hypertension. The frequency of renal vascular hypertension may be as high as 33 percent in such patients (see Section #5).

Women Taking Oral Contraceptives

After starting estrogen-containing oral contraceptives, most women experience a 2 to 4 mm Hg increase in blood pressure. As many as five percent of previously normotensive women will have a rise of DBP above 90 mm Hg after five years of pill use, a rate two to three times higher than women not taking the pill. The reason blood pressure rises more in some women is unknown, but they may have a pre-existing propensity to develop primary hypertension or underlying renal dysfunction (see Section #7).

Children

Pre-pubertal hypertensive children most likely have a renal cause. Post-pubertal children most likely have primary hypertension but a higher frequency of certain secondary causes is seen among them (see Section #30).

Elderly

Those who have the onset of hypertension after age 50, and even more so after age 60, have a higher frequency of renal parenchymal disease and renovascular hypertension.

References

Choudhri AH, et al: Unsuspected renal artery stenosis in peripheral vascular disease. Br Med J 1990;301:1197-1198.

Danielson M, Dammstrom B-G: The prevalence of secondary and curable hypertension. Acta Med Scand 1981;209:451-455.

Lewin A, et al: Apparent prevalence of curable hypertension in the Hypertension Detection and Follow-up Program. Arch Intern Med 1985;145:424-427.

Sinclair AM, et al: Secondary hypertension in a blood pressure clinic. Arch Intern Med 1987;147:1289-1293.

#4 Primary Hypertension

Background

The specific cause of primary hypertension is unknown (Figure 4.1). A genetic predisposition has been documented with about a two-fold higher incidence in those with a close relative who is hypertensive. Environmental factors which increase the incidence include:

- Obesity, particularly upper body
- Psychogenic stress
- High sodium intake
- Alcohol intake greater than one ounce per day

Blood pressure may rise as a consequence of an increase in either cardiac output or peripheral resistance (Figure 4.2). Although cardiac output may be high initially, hypertension usually persists because of increased peripheral resistance. This, in turn, may arise from both functional tightening and structural thickening of resistance vessels. Multiple factors may be responsible. Resistance to the actions of insulin on peripheral muscles has been shown in hypertensives and the resultant hyperinsulinemia may serve as a stimulus for vascular hypertrophy.

The disease usually:

- Appears between ages 30 and 50
- Is slowly progressive
- Remains asymptomatic until significant target organ damage appears after 10 to 20 years

Evaluation

For the majority of adult and adolescent hypertensive patients, the following evaluation should be done to assess target organ damage, to rule out secondary causes and to ascertain the overall cardiovascular risk status:

- Hematocrit
- Urine analysis
- Automated blood chemistry
  - Creatinine
  - Fasting glucose
  - Sodium

FIGURE 4.1 – Natural History of Untreated Primary Hypertension

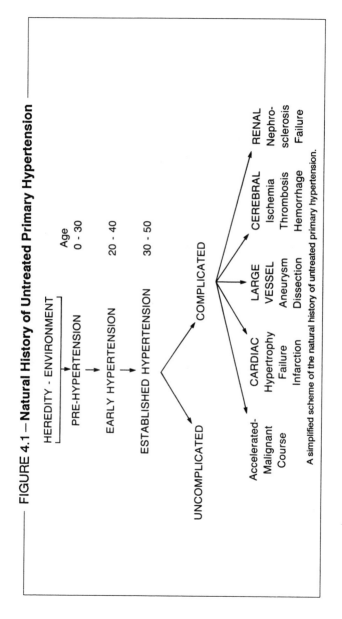

A simplified scheme of the natural history of untreated primary hypertension.

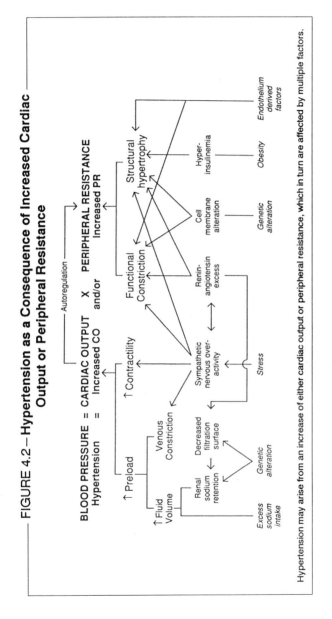

FIGURE 4.2 – Hypertension as a Consequence of Increased Cardiac Output or Peripheral Resistance

BLOOD PRESSURE = CARDIAC OUTPUT X PERIPHERAL RESISTANCE
Hypertension = Increased CO and/or Increased PR

Hypertension may arise from an increase of either cardiac output or peripheral resistance, which in turn are affected by multiple factors.

20

- Potassium
- Total cholesterol
- HDL-cholesterol
- Electrocardiogram

Additional tests may be needed for those in the previously noted special populations or who display suggestive features of a secondary cause by history or physical examination (Table 4.1).

In the near future, two additional procedures may be more frequently indicated, since current evidence shows that they are more sensitive indices of the severity of hypertension: echocardiography, which shows left ventricular hypertrophy much earlier than electrocardiography, and 24-hour ambulatory blood pressure monitoring, which has been found to predict the development of target organ damage more accurately than by the levels obtained by repeated office measurements.

TABLE 4.1 ➤

TABLE 4.1 – Overall Guides for Evaluation

Diagnostic Procedure

Diagnosis	Initial	Additional
Chronic renal disease	Urinalysis, BUN or creatinine, sonography	Renin assay, renal biopsy, IVP
Renovascular disease	Bruit, plasma renin before and one hour after 25 mg captopril	Aortogram, renal vein renins
Coarctation	Blood pressure in legs	Aortogram
Primary aldosteronism	Plasma potassium	Urinary potassium, plasma renin, plasma or urinary aldosterone
Cushing's syndrome	A.M. plasma cortisol after 1 mg dexamethasone at bedtime	Urinary cortisol after variable doses of dexamethasone
Pheochromocytoma	Spot urine for metanephrine	Urinary metanephrine and catechols; plasma catechols, basal and after 0.3 mg clonidine

References

Biron P, Mongeau JG, Bertrand D: Familial aggregation of blood pressure in 588 adopted children. Canad Med Assoc J 1976;155:773- 776.

Brigden G, et al: Effects of noninvasive ambulatory blood pressure measuring devices on blood pressure. Am J Cardiol 1990;66:1396-1398.

Julius S, et al: Hyperkinetic borderline hypertension in Tecumseh, Michigan. J Hypertension 1991;9:77-84.

Kaplan NM: The deadly quartet: Upper-body obesity, glucose intolerance, hypertriglyceridemia, and hypertension. Arch Intern Med 1989;149:1514-1520.

Khaw K-T, Barrett-Connor E: The association between blood pressure, age, and dietary sodium and potassium: A population study. Circulation 1988;77:53-61.

Natali A, et al: Impaired insulin action on skeletal muscle metabolism in essential hypertension. Hypertension 1991;17: 170-178.

Pearson AC, Pasierski T, Labovitz AJ: Left ventricular hypertrophy: Diagnosis, prognosis, and management. Am Heart J 1991;121:148-157.

Pollare T, Lithell H, Berne C: Insulin resistance is a characteristic feature of primary hypertension independent of obesity. Metabolism 1990;39:167-174.

Sealey JE, et al: On the renal basis for essential hypertension: Nephron heterogeneity with discordant renin secretion and sodium excretion causing a hypertensive vasoconstriction-volume relationship. J Hypertens 1988;6:763-777.

Strazzullo P, et al: Altered extracellular calcium homeostasis in essential hypertension: A consequence of abnormal cell calcium handling. Clin Sci 1986;71:239-244.

Trevisan M, et al: Red blood cell Na content, Na, Li-counter-transport, family history of hypertension, and blood pressure in school children. J Hypertens 1988;6:227-230.

#5 Secondary Hypertension: Renal

Renal Parenchymal Disease
Renal Vascular Hypertension

Frequency

Beyond obesity, oral contraceptive use in women, and alcohol abuse in men, renal parenchymal and vascular diseases are the most common causes of secondary hypertension, particularly in children, the elderly and those with severe or resistant disease.

RENAL PARENCHYMAL DISEASE

A considerable percentage of patients, as many as 10 percent, who start with primary hypertension develop progressive nephrosclerosis and end up with chronic renal failure. This course is more common among black hypertensives and those who have co-existing diabetes mellitus or poorly controlled hypertension.

As renal function deteriorates, hypertension becomes more prevalent and is present in about 85 percent of those with end-stage renal disease (ESRD). In such patients, it may not be possible to dissect cause from effect but renal function is normal in most with primary hypertension whose blood pressure is well controlled, whereas renal dysfunction (proteinuria, elevated serum creatinine, lower GFR) is prominent even without significant hypertension in most with a renal cause.

Clinical Features

The blood pressures tend to rise as renal function is lost, mainly from the inability of the damaged kidneys to excrete sodium and water. In some, renin hypersecretion is responsible and the absence of normal renal vasodepressor hormones may be involved.

All forms of progressive renal disease may lead to hypertension, including:
- Polycystic disease (frequently)
- Analgesic nephropathy (less frequently)

- Vasculitis (as in collagen vascular disease, may induce acute, severe, renal failure)
- Pyelonephritis (rarely, except in patients with reflux nephropathy)
- Diabetic nephropathy (becoming more prevalent as more patients with diabetes live for 20 years or longer after developing the disease)

Management

The effective control of hypertension may slow and even partially reverse the progress of renal failure. Control may be accomplished by:
- Reduction in fluid volume by restriction of dietary sodium
- High doses of loop diuretics
- Dialysis

More potent antihypertensive agents, in particular minoxidil, may be especially useful (see Section #33). In experimental models, converting enzyme inhibitors and calcium-entry blockers provide special protection against progression of renal damage.

RENAL VASCULAR HYPERTENSION

Clinical Features

In most patients with renal vascular hypertension (RVH), one or more of these features will be noted:
- Onset of hypertension before age 30 or after age 50
- Rapid progression of the degree of hypertension
- A diastolic bruit lateral to the midline, just below the rib cage in the mid-epigastrium
- Poor response to most antihypertensive drugs
- Rapid progression of renal insufficiency after use of an angiotensin-converting enzyme (ACE) inhibitor usually heralds bilateral renal hypertension or stenosis of the artery to a solitary kidney. In both settings, the renal circulation is critically dependent on high levels of angiotensin II (A-II). A-II levels are lowered by the ACE inhibitor and renal blood flow is markedly reduced

In the younger, particularly women, medial fibroplasia is the most common form of renal vascular disease. In the older, atherosclerotic plaques are most common.

Diagnosis

In some, renovascular hypertension cannot be distinguished on clinical grounds from primary hypertension. Nothing is lost if the diagnosis is not made in such patients, as long as their hypertension can be well controlled and usual indices of renal function (serum creatinine) remain normal.

Those with the suggestive features listed above should be evaluated for RVH. The more suggestive the features, the more essential it is to do the definitive diagnostic test, a renal arteriogram. The use of digital subtraction equipment makes arteriography safe enough to be done as an outpatient procedure, except in diabetics. Renal vein ratios may be useful to establish the diagnosis, but intravenous pyelography and digital subtraction venous angiography have little place in the evaluation. Plasma renin levels 60 minutes after 50 mg of captopril may be the easiest screening procedure, as described by Muller, et al.

Therapy

Medical therapy, even if successful in control of hypertension, may not stop the progress of renal atrophy. Surgical repair is preferable, particularly in younger patients. Percutaneous angioplasty has been used increasingly as initial therapy, particularly in poor surgical candidates. However, lasting relief of hypertension has been obtained in only about one-third of patients. The procedure may be repeated in those who respond but in whom hypertension recurs.

References

Anderson S, et al: Control of glomerular hypertension limits glomerular injury in rats with reduced renal mass. J Clin Invest 1985;76:612-619.

Fine LG: Preventing the progression of human renal disease: Have rational therapeutic principles emerged? Kidney Int 1988;33:116-128.

Frederickson ED, et al: A prospective evaluation of a simplified captopril test for the detection of renovascular hypertension. Arch Intern Med 1990;150:569-572.

Hurwitz GA, et al: Screening for a renovascular etiology in hypertensive patients undergoing myocardial scintigraphy: Differential renal thallium-201 uptake. Can J Cardiol 1990; 6:198-204.

Kalra PA, et al: Renovascular disease and renal complications of angiotensin-converting enzyme inhibitor therapy. Q J Med 1990;77:1013-1018.

Kaylor WM, et al: Reversal of end stage renal failure with surgical revascularization in patients with atherosclerotic renal artery occlusion. J Urol 1989;141:486-488.

Luscher TF, et al: Curable renal parenchymatous hypertension: Current diagnosis and management. Cardiol 1985; 72(Suppl 1):33-45.

Muller FB, et al: The captopril test for identifying renovascular disease in hypertensive patients. Am J Med 1986;80:633-644.

Ramsay LE, Waller PC: Blood pressure response to percutaneous transluminal angioplasty for renovascular hypertension: An overview of published series. Br Med J 1990;300:569-572.

Ying CY, et al: Renal revascularization in the azotemic hypertensive patient resistant to therapy. N Engl J Med 1984; 311:1070-1075.

#6 Secondary Hypertension: Adrenal

Pheochromocytoma
Cushing's Syndrome
Primary Aldosteronism

Types of Adrenal Hypertension

Hypertension accompanies hyperfunction of the adrenal medulla (pheochromocytoma) or cortex (Cushing's syndrome from excess cortisol or primary aldosteronism). In total, these syndromes comprise less than one percent of hypertension among adults. In children, hypersecretion of mineralocorticoids can be the consequence of congenital adrenal enzyme deficiencies (congenital adrenal hyperplasia).

PHEOCHROMOCYTOMA

Clinical Features

The types and approximate frequency of occurrence of the tumors are:

- Unilateral, benign (80 percent)
- Malignant (10 percent)
- Bilateral, benign (10 percent)

Bilateral benign tumors are often part of the multiple endocrine adenoma (MEA) syndrome accompanied by medullary cancer of the thyroid.

The hypertension may be episodic or sustained, but intermittent "spells" are almost always noted that include:

- Headache
- Tachycardia
- Sweating
- Tremor

The excess catecholamines usually induce a hypermetabolic state with:

- Weight loss
- Hyperglycemia
- Intense peripheral vasoconstriction with paleness

Diagnosis

Patients with widely fluctuating blood pressure and repeated "spells" should have a spot urine analyzed for metanephrine as a screening test. If the spot urine metanephrine is above 1.0 microgram per mg creatinine, a 24 hour urine should be analyzed for metanephrine and catecholamines. Further documentation may be obtained by measurement of plasma catecholamines, first with the patient in a basal state and then three hours after 0.3 mg of clonidine which will suppress catecholamine secretion from normal adrenals but not from pheochromocytomas.

An abdominal CT scan will usually demonstrate the tumor. MIBG isotopic scans may be used for those not identified by CT.

Therapy

Surgery should be performed after the manifestations of catecholamine excess are reversed by alpha-receptor blockade, preferably with dibenzyline or prazosin and, if tachycardia is prominent, the addition of a beta-blocker.

CUSHING'S SYNDROME

Clinical Features

Hypertension is present in approximately 85 percent of patients with Cushing's syndrome whether it is caused by:
- Bilateral adrenal hyperplasia from ACTH hypersecretion from the pituitary or an ectopic tumor
- A benign adrenal tumor
- An adrenal carcinoma

Cortisol excess is usually manifested by:
- Redistribution of body fat (truncal obesity)
- Decrease in protein synthesis (thin skin with striae and ecchymoses, osteoporosis)
- Increase in glucose synthesis (hyperglycemia)

Diagnosis

Measurement of plasma cortisol obtained the morning after a 1 mg dose of dexamethasone at bedtime is an excellent screening test, with almost all non-Cushing's patients suppressing below 7 microgram/dL. Documentation of the type of Cushing's can be made by more prolonged administration of varying doses of dexamethasone, measuring 24 hour urine cortisol levels. Plasma ACTH levels and CT scans will provide additional confirmation of the type of Cushing's and may supplant the prolonged dexamethasone suppression tests.

Therapy

The cause of the cortisol excess, either from the pituitary in those with bilateral hyperplasia or from an adrenal tumor, should be surgically removed. Various inhibitors of cortisol synthesis are available to prepare for surgery or to provide at least partial control for those in whom surgery is not feasible.

PRIMARY ALDOSTERONISM

Clinical Features

Mineralocorticoid excess may arise from a solitary benign adenoma or bilateral hyperplasia. In general, secretion is greater from an adenoma so the manifestations are more severe:

- Plasma potassium is lower
- Plasma renin activity is lower
- Plasma and urine aldosterone is higher

The syndrome should be considered in hypertensives with hypokalemia that is not provoked by diuretics, GI losses, etc. Almost all patients will have hypertension, which is often severe in degree, and hypokalemia, which may be intermittent (Figure 6.1).

Diagnosis

The finding of urinary potassium wastage of more than 30 mmol/day in the face of low plasma K+ is a useful initial screening test if the urine is collected without

FIGURE 6.1 – The Pathophysiology of Primary Aldosteronism

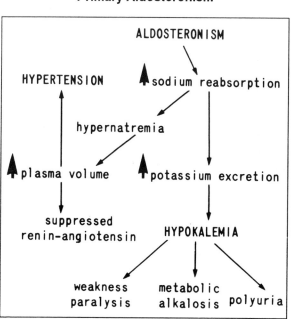

The pathophysiology of primary aldosteronism (From Kaplan NM. *Clinical Hypertension*. *5th ed.*, Baltimore: Williams & Wilkins, 1990.)

sodium restriction or potassium supplementation. If a blood sample obtained after recognition of hypokalemia contains high aldosterone (above 20 ng/dL) and low renin activity (below 1 ng/mL/hr), primary aldosteronism is likely. Autonomous hypersecretion of aldosterone may be demonstrated by failure to suppress plasma aldosterone below 6 ng/dL after 2 liters of IV normal saline over four hours. CT scans will usually demonstrate the adrenal pathology but a number of special procedures may be needed for additional confirmation if a tumor is not seen.

Therapy

Adenomas should be surgically removed. Bilateral hyperplasia should be controlled with the aldosterone antagonist spironolactone. If that is poorly tolerated, amiloride or triamterene will usually correct the hypokalemia. A thiazide diuretic may also be needed.

Apparent Mineralocorticoid Excess

Apparent mineralocorticoid excess (ie, hypertension, hypokalemia, but low levels of aldosterone) can be induced by inhibition of the $11\text{-}\beta$-hydroxysteroid dehydrogenase enzyme that normally converts cortisol (which binds to the renal mineralocorticoid receptor) to cortisone (which does not bind). The persistent high level of cortisol in the kidney acts as a potent mineralocorticoid. The glycyrrhizic acid present in licorice (now frequently added to chewing tobacco) will inhibit the enzyme and induce the syndrome.

References

Bravo EL, et al: Clinical implications of primary aldosteronism with resistant hypertension. Hypertension 1988;11(Suppl I): I-207-211.

Irony I, et al: Correctable subsets of primary aldosteronism. Primary adrenal hyperplasia and renin responsive adenoma. Am J Hypertens 1990;3:576-82.

Jeffcoate WJ: Treating Cushing's disease. Br Med J 1988;296: 227-228.

Kennedy L, et al: Serum cortisol concentrations during low dose dexamethasone suppression test to screen for Cushing's syndrome. Br Med J 1984;289:1188-1191.

Ross EJ, Linch DC: Cushing's syndrome—killing disease: Discriminatory value of signs and symptoms aiding early diagnosis. Lancet 1982;2:646-649.

Sheps SG, et al: Recent developments in the diagnosis and treatment of pheochromocytoma. Mayo Clin Proc 1990;65:88-95.

Sonino N: The use of ketoconazole as an inhibitor of steroid production. N Engl J Med 1987;317:812-818.

Stewart PM, et al: Syndrome of apparent mineralocorticoid excess. A defect in the cortisol-cortisone shuttle. J Clin Invest 1988;82:340-349.

Stockigt JR, Scoggins BA: Long-term evolution of glucocorticoid-suppressible hyperaldosteronism. J Clin Endocrinol Metab 1986;64:22-26.

Young WF Jr, et al: Primary aldosteronism: Diagnosis and treatment. Mayo Clin Proc 1990;65:96-110.

#7 Secondary Hypertension: Estrogen and Pregnancy

Estrogen-Induced Hypertension
Pregnancy Hypertension

Clinical Information

As many as five percent of women who take estrogen-containing oral contraceptives (OCs) and a somewhat smaller percentage of pregnant women will develop reversible hypertension. The former contributes to the vascular complications of OCs, the latter is a major cause of fetal mortality.

7.

ESTROGEN-INDUCED HYPERTENSION

Clinical Features

Although the use of estrogens as postmenopausal replacement therapy does not lead to hypertension, their use in the form of oral contraceptives may do so.

The blood pressure rises a few mm Hg in most who take estrogen-containing OCs. About five percent will rise beyond 140/90 within five years. If the OC is stopped, hypertension will recede in about two-thirds of this five percent. The remaining one-third will either have underlying primary hypertension or have suffered vascular damage that sustains the OC-induced rise in blood pressure.

The hypertension is usually mild but rarely may induce severe renal vascular damage. The mechanism for the hypertension is uncertain but may involve estrogen-induced increases in renin substrate that somehow cause increased angiotensin II levels. Less hypertension may accompany the use of OCs with low content of estrogen.

Management

Women over age 35 should not use OCs, particularly if they smoke cigarettes. When used for temporary birth control in younger women, they are quite safe. The blood pressure should be monitored every three to six months. If hypertension develops, another form of contraception should be substituted.

PREGNANCY HYPERTENSION

Clinical Features

During pregnancy, hypertension may be noted early, when it usually represents primary hypertension, or late, when it usually represents the self-limited process, pregnancy-induced hypertension (PIH). The latter, if accompanied by proteinuria and edema, is usually called preeclampsia; if encephalopathy and convulsions ensue, the process is called eclampsia.

In response to vasodilation, the blood pressure normally falls during the first and second trimesters, with levels of 100/60 commonly noted. Women who have unrecognized hypertension before pregnancy may lower their high levels enough to be no longer hypertensive. When their levels rise during the later months, they may be thought to have PIH, the self-limited disease that arises during the last trimester and disappears soon after delivery. Edema and proteinuria usually occur with PIH.

Most self-limited PIH occurs in the last few weeks of pregnancy. The majority of women with hypertension appearing before week 36 have underlying (previous) essential hypertension or renal disease.

The diagnosis of PIH has been based on a rise of more than 30/15 mm Hg or to a level above 140/90 in the last half of pregnancy. To reduce the number of misdiagnoses of chronic hypertension as PIH, the diastolic blood pressure should have been measured earlier as below 90 mm Hg but risen at least 25 mm Hg to above 90.

Mechanisms

PIH is most likely to appear among:
- Young primigravidae
- Those with underlying vascular disease (diabetes, primary hypertension)
- Those with large placental mass (multiple births, moles)

These associations have suggested that the process is induced by reduced uteroplacental blood flow. Hemodynamically, the vascular bed is constricted. The vasoconstriction has been attributed to both increased levels of renin-angiotensin and reduced levels of vasodilatory prostaglandins, perhaps associated with an excess of vasoconstricting thromboxanes. The role of prostaglandin imbalance, arising perhaps from disordered placental steroid synthesis, has been supported by reports of a reduced incidence of PIH among women considered to be susceptible who were given 60 mg of aspirin per day. Large scale preventative trials with low doses of aspirin are in progress.

Management

Women diagnosed as having PIH should restrict activity and be carefully monitored, preferably in a high-risk pregnancy unit. Antihypertensives are given only if DBP remains above 100 mg Hg and diuretics are used only if congestive heart failure supervenes.

Women with chronic hypertension have been successfully managed with methyldopa and, more recently, beta-blockers. However, small fetal size has been reported after beta-blocker use.

If eclampsia threatens, parenteral magnesium is used as an anticonvulsant. The overall aim of management is to allow the fetus to reach adequate maturity while protecting the mother from vascular damage.

References

Butters L, Kennedy S, Rubin PC: Atenolol in essential hypertension during pregnancy. Br Med J 1990:301:587-589.

Constantine G, et al: Nifedipine as a second line antihypertensive drug in pregnancy. Br J Obstet Gynecol 1987;94:1136-1142.

Fitzgerald DJ, et al: Thromboxane A_2 synthesis in pregnancy-induced hypertension. Lancet 1990;335:751-754.

Gallery ED, Ross MR, Gyory AZ: Antihypertensive treatment in pregnancy: Analysis of different responses to oxprenolol and methyldopa. Br Med J 1985;291:563-566.

National High Blood Pressure Education Program Working Group report on high blood pressure in pregnancy. Am J Obstet Gynecol 1990;163:1689-1712.

Redman CWG, Jefferies M: Revised definition of pre-eclampsia. Lancet 1988;1:809-812.

Schiff E, et al: The use of aspirin to prevent pregnancy-induced hypertension and lower the ratio of thromboxane A_2 to prostacyclin in relatively high risk pregnancies. N Engl J Med 1989; 321:351-356.

Wallenberg HCS, et al: Low-dose aspirin prevents pregnancy-induced hypertension and pre-eclampsia in angiotensin-sensitive primigravidae. Lancet 1986;1:1-3.

Woods JW: Oral contraceptives and hypertension. Hypertension 1988;11(Suppl II):II-11-15.

#8 Secondary Hypertension: Other Causes

Hormonal
Stress/Surgery
Neurogenic

Clinical Information

The large number of relatively rare forms of secondary hypertension infrequently pose either diagnostic or therapeutic difficulty. The following covers only the more common or potentially serious forms.

HORMONAL

Hyperparathyroidism

Hypercalcemia from any cause may increase peripheral resistance and raise the blood pressure. Most patients with hyperparathyroidism are hypertensive, although the blood pressure becomes normal only in a minority after cure of the hyperparathyroidism.

Hypothyroidism

The diastolic blood pressure may be increased from peripheral vasoconstriction but the systolic level is usually not increased since cardiac output is reduced.

Hyperthyroidism

The high cardiac output tends to raise systolic levels but the diastolic is usually reduced, presumably because of peripheral vasodilation in response to increased metabolic demands.

Acromegaly

Most patients are hypertensive, likely as a result of fluid volume excess.

Acute Stress and Anxiety

Marked activation of the sympathetic nervous system may induce considerable hypertension. Patients with severe chest pain from myocardial ischemia or abdominal pain from acute pancreatitis usually have significant hypertension which may rapidly recede as the pain is relieved. Caution should be taken in using potent parenteral antihypertensive agents in such patients unless their high pressures remain a threat after relief of their acute symptoms.

Transient elevations in pressure may accompany anxiety-induced acute hyperventilation.

Postoperative

Blood pressure may rise during and after surgery in response to various stimuli, including:

- Hypoxia
- Pain
- Volume excess

A particularly high frequency of hypertension follows coronary bypass surgery, likely as a result of marked sympathetic nervous stimulation. Surgery on the carotid arteries may also be followed by significant hypertension.

Various parenteral antihypertensive agents have been used to treat perioperative hypertension. Nitroprusside is most potent but cumbersome to use; labetalol, nicardipine or esmolol may be effective alternatives.

Burns

Many with third-degree burns over more than 20 percent of body surface will develop hypertension which may require appropriate therapy.

NEUROGENIC

Sleep Apnea

A significant percentage of hypertensive patients have sleep apnea, particularly if they are overweight. In most, the apnea is obstructive rather than central and therefore has been assumed to be the cause of the hypertension rather than a consequence of CNS damage. Relief of airway obstruction has been shown to result in lowering of blood pressure.

Drugs

Cyclosporine

As many as half of patients given this immunosuppressive drug will develop hypertension, even in the absence of renal damage.

Sympathomimetic

Street drugs (amphetamines, cocaine) and over-the-counter drugs (phenylpropanolamine, pseudoephedrine) may induce considerable hypertension.

Nonsteroidal Anti-Inflammatory Agents

Presumably by decreasing vasodilatory prostaglandins, these drugs may interfere with the efficacy of various antihypertensive drugs.

Increased Intracranial Pressure

Significant hypertension can be caused by:
- Brain tumors
- Acute strokes
- Head trauma

It is presumably a result of irritation of vasomotor centers or disruptions of sympathetic nervous control.

Hypoglycemia

The catecholamine response to insulin-induced hypoglycemia may provoke severe hypertension, particularly in patients receiving beta-blockers.

References

Bravo EL: Phenylpropanolamine and other over-the-counter vasoactive compounds. Hypertension 1988;11(Suppl II):II-7-10.

Brown J, Dollery C, Valdes G: Interaction of nonsteroidal anti-inflammatory drugs with antihypertensive and diuretic agents. Control of vascular reactivity by endogenous prostanoids. Am J Med 1986;81(Suppl 2B):43-57.

Cooper TJ, et al: Factors relating to the development of hypertension after cardiopulmonary bypass. Br Heart J 1985;54:91-95.

Daniels J, Goodman AD: Hypertension and hyperparathyroidism: Inverse relation of serum phosphate level and blood pressure. Am J Med 1983;75:17-23.

Fyman PN, et al: Vasodilator therapy in the perioperative period. Can Anaesth Soc J 1986;33:629-643.

Mihatsch MJ, et al: Cyclosporin-associated nephropathy in patients with autoimmune diseases. Clin Wochenschr 1988;66:43-47.

Stradling JR, Crosby JH: Relation between systemic hypertension and sleep hypoxaemia or snoring: Analysis in 748 men drawn from general practice. Br Med J 1990;300:75-78.

Streeten DHP, et al: Effects of thyroid function on blood pressure. Recognition of hypothyroid hypertension. Hypertension 1988;11:78-83.

#9 Non-Drug Therapy: Dietary

Weight Reduction
Sodium Restriction
Other Dietary Changes

Clinical Information

Once hypertension is diagnosed and the patient evaluated, therapy should be provided. For many, therapy will include antihypertensive drugs. Issues concerning the decision to use drugs are included in Section #11 and specifics about the various agents are included in other sections. Whether drugs are used, a variety of non-drug therapies should be offered to all patients with any degree of hypertension. Those involving the diet will be included in this section. Other non-drug therapies are covered in Section #10.

WEIGHT REDUCTION

9.

Almost half of all hypertensive people are over-weight. As weight is gained, the blood pressure tends to rise; if weight is lost, the blood pressure usually falls. Sleep apnea may be involved in a larger segment of the obese hypertensive population than now recognized. Studies have shown that 30 percent or more of even slightly obese hypertensives have sleep apnea and in some the hypertension may recede when the sleep apnea is overcome.

Hyperinsulinemia is present in obese people, particularly in those whose obesity is predominantly in the abdomen and upper body. High levels of insulin may raise the blood pressure by multiple mechanisms.

Calories should be restricted in a manner appropriate to the individual patient. For most, a 1,200 calorie low-fat diet will provide gradual weight loss without discomfort. For some, more restrictive diets may be needed, such as the substitution of a 400 to 600 calorie per day, high quality protein-powder with appropriate electrolyte and vitamin supplement.

SODIUM RESTRICTION

Restriction of dietary sodium to 2 g per day (88 mmol or 5 g of NaCl) will lower the blood pressure by 5 to 10 mm Hg in a significant number of "sodium-sensitive" hypertensives. This degree of restriction can be attained by avoiding highly salted foods, eg, pickles, processed meats, sauerkraut and adding no salt at the table or in the cooking. KCl may be used as a salt substitute, either alone or with NaCl, with caution in those with renal insufficiency.

An awareness is required of the "hidden" sodium present in most processed foods such as canned vegetables and many breakfast cereals (Table 9.1). Fresh or unprocessed frozen foods should be used whenever possible.

Although not all patients will respond to such moderate sodium restriction, no harm should occur from the return to the natural lower-sodium diet consumed by humans throughout history until the recent past. The reduction in sodium may reduce potassium loss if diuretics are given and the lower-sodium fresh foods will likely have higher amounts of potassium than are present in their processed forms.

More rigid sodium restriction may be needed for patients with renal failure or severe heart failure. If needed, low-sodium preparations of a number of processed foods are available.

OTHER DIETARY CHANGES

Potassium Supplementation

Correction of hypokalemia may lower the blood pressure. Although supplemental KCl has been shown to lower the blood pressure in some normokalemic hypertensives, there should be little need to give such supplements if natural, high-potassium foods are substituted for processed, high-sodium foods in the diet. Supplements of KCl may be required to replenish potassium deficiency since dietary sources of potassium may be largely accompanied by non-reabsorbable anions which reduce retention of the potassium.

TABLE 9.1 – The Sodium Content of Some Common Foods
(1,000 mg Sodium = 44 mEq Sodium)

**Comparable foods with either low
or high sodium content**

Low

Shredded Wheat	1 mg/oz
Green beans, fresh	5 mg/cup
Orange juice	2 mg/cup
Turkey, roasted	70 mg/3-oz
Ground beef	57 mg/3-oz
Pork, uncooked	65 mg/3-oz

High

Corn Flakes	305 mg/oz
Green beans, canned	925 mg/cup
Tomato juice	640 mg/cup
Turkey dinner	1,735 mg
Frankfurter, beef	425 mg each
Bacon, uncooked	1,400 mg/3-oz

Sodium content of some "Fast Foods"

Kentucky Fried Chicken (three pieces of chicken, potatoes, gravy, coleslaw and roll)	2,285 mg
McDonald's Big Mac	962 mg
Burger King Whopper	909 mg
Dairy Queen chili dog	939 mg
Taco Bell enchirito	1,175 mg

Some foods with very high sodium content

Catsup, one tablespoon	156 mg
Olive, one	165 mg
Cinnamon roll, one	630 mg
Soup (chicken noodle), one cup	1,050 mg
Dill pickle, one large	1,928 mg

Calcium Supplementation

In a few patients, 1 to 2 g of supplemental calcium per day has been found to lower blood pressure. These patients may be those with hypercalcinuria which, by reducing serum ionized calcium levels, may raise blood parathyroid hormone, which in turn may further raise blood pressure. Even though supplemental calcium may reduce their blood pressure, hypercalcinuria may worsen.

Magnesium Supplementation

Magnesium supplements have not usually been noted to lower blood pressure. However, patients who are deficient in both magnesium and potassium may not be able to replete potassium stores unless magnesium is also provided.

Lower Fat, Higher Fiber

A few well-controlled studies have shown that the intake of a lower saturated, higher unsaturated fat diet will reduce the blood pressure. The effect may be attributable to an increase in synthesis of vasodilatory prostaglandins.

One study has shown a fall in blood pressure with a high fiber diet.

Moderation of Alcohol

Besides adding calories, alcohol consumption may raise the blood pressure. One ounce of alcohol per day will likely not raise the blood pressure, but will provide protection against coronary heart disease (CHD) and mortality. This can be in the form of either:
- Two beers
- Two glasses of wine
- Two mixed drinks

This has been demonstrated in many epidemiological surveys wherein those who drink one ounce of ethanol per day have less CHD than those who do not drink ethanol.

However, in multiple population surveys, daily consumption of more than one ounce of alcohol per day is associated with higher blood pressure and more than two ounces per day is often associated with overt hypertension.

References

Cappuccio FP, et al: Lack of effect of oral magnesium on high blood pressure: A double blind study. Br Med J 1985;291:235-238.

Cutler JA, Brittain E: Calcium and blood pressure: An epidemiologic perspective. Am J Hypertens 1990;3:137S-146S.

Fodor JG, Chockalingam A: The Canadian Consensus Report on Non-Pharmacological Approaches to the Management of High Blood Pressure. Clin Exper Hyper 1990;A12:729-743.

Fukagawa NK, et al: High-carbohydrate, high-fiber diets increase peripheral insulin sensitivity in healthy young and old adults. Am J Clin Nutr 1990;52:524-528.

Grimm RH Jr, et al: The influence of oral potassium chloride on blood pressure in hypertensive men on a low-sodium diet. N Engl J Med 1990;322:569-574.

Kaplan NM, et al: Potassium supplementation in hypertensive patients with diuretic-induced hypokalemia. N Engl J Med 1985;312:746-749.

Kaplan NM, Meese RB: The calcium deficiency hypothesis of hypertension: A critique. Ann Intern Med 1986;105:947-955.

Parker M, et al: Two-way factorial study of alcohol and salt restriction in treated hypertensive men. Hypertension 1990; 16:398-406.

Reaven GM, Hoffman BB: A role for insulin in the aetiology and course of hypertension? Lancet 1987;2:434-436.

Staessen J, et al: Body weight, sodium intake and blood pressure. J Hypertension 1989;7(Suppl 1):S12-S23.

Working Group on Management of Patients with Hypertension and High Blood Cholesterol. National Education Programs Working Group report on the management of patients with hypertension and high blood cholesterol. Ann Intern Med 1991;114:224-237.

#10 Non-Drug Therapy: Other

Isotonic Exercise
Relaxation Therapy
Overall Non-Drug Program

Clinical Information

Beyond dietary changes, other non-drug therapies may help lower the blood pressure. These include isotonic exercise and one or another form of relaxation therapy. Claims have been made for other modalities as varied as garlic and acupuncture but their efficacy has not been shown in properly controlled clinical trials.

ISOTONIC EXERCISE

A number of studies have shown that regular isotonic (dynamic or aerobic) exercise is accompanied by a fall in blood pressure. Although some of the antihypertensive effects of exercise may reflect coincidental weight loss, changes in diet, etc., hypertensives should be encouraged to perform regular isotonic exercises.

The form of exercise is irrelevant as long as it is isotonic, ie, involves active movement of muscles. During isotonic exercise, cardiac output rises but peripheral resistance falls from vasodilation in muscle vasculature. Systolic blood pressure rises but diastolic pressure tends to fall or remain the same. Isometric exercise, ie, increased tension without movement, is associated with a reflex increase in both cardiac output and peripheral resistance, causing marked rises in both systolic and diastolic blood pressure while the isometric exercise is being performed.

Some normotensive people have marked increases in systolic blood pressure, beyond 180 mm Hg, during the intense exercise of a stress test. Preliminary data suggests that such people may have a somewhat higher likelihood of subsequently developing permanent hypertension but this is by no means invariable.

10

To reach the "conditioned" state of cardiac performance, 20 to 30 minutes of sustained exercise at 70 percent of maximal capacity, usually determined from the rise in pulse rate, is required three times each week. The level of exercise that accomplishes the greatest fall in blood pressure has not been determined.

RELAXATION THERAPY

Almost all forms of relaxation therapy have been said to lower the blood pressure. These include:
- Progressive muscle relaxation
- Yoga
- Biofeedback
- Transcendental meditation
- The Chinese breathing exercise Qi Gong
- Hypnosis

Only a few controlled studies have shown a sustained effect beyond the duration of the relaxation procedure. Those patients who are willing to continue the practice of one or another relaxation therapy should be encouraged to do so.

OVERALL NON-DRUG PROGRAM

The steps which should be followed as part of an overall non-drug program include:
- Reduce excess body weight by caloric restriction. Caution against the use of over-the-counter appetite suppressants—most contain sympathomimetics which may raise the blood pressure
- Restrict dietary sodium to 2 g per day (88 mmol or 5 g of NaCl), about half the amount in the usual North American diet
- Reduce dietary saturated fat and cholesterol
- Maintain adequate intake of potassium, calcium and magnesium, supplementing those who are deficient

- Limit alcohol intake to no more than two ounces and preferably one ounce per day (one ounce of alcohol contained in two usual portions of beer, wine or spirits)
- Perform 20 to 30 minutes of isotonic exercise at least three times a week
- Use whatever form of relaxation therapy that is acceptable
- Stop smoking. This will probably not influence the blood pressure but will have a powerfully beneficial effect on overall cardiovascular health

References

Chesney MA, Black GW: Behavioral treatment of borderline hypertension: An overview of results. J Cardiovasc Pharmacol 1986;8(Suppl 5);S57-S63.

Duncan JJ, et al: The effects of aerobic exercise on plasma catecholamines and blood pressure in patients with mild essential hypertension. JAMA 1985;254:2609-2613.

Ehsani AA, et al: Exercise training improves left ventricular systolic function in older men. Circulation 1991;83:96-103.

Health and Public Policy Committee: Biofeedback for hypertension. Ann Intern Med 1985;102:709-715.

Jennings G, et al: The effects of changes in physical activity on major cardiovascular risk factors, hemodynamics, sympathetic function, and glucose utilization in man. Circulation 1986;73:30-40.

Kelemen MH, et al: Exercise training combined with antihypertensive drug therapy. JAMA 1990;263:2766-2771.

Patel C, Marmot M: Can general practitioners use training in relaxation and management of stress to reduce mild hypertension? Br Med J 1988;296:21-24.

Stamler R, et al: Primary prevention of hypertension by nutritional-hygienic means. Final report of a randomized, controlled trial. JAMA 1989;262:1801-1807.

#11 The Decision to Use Drugs

Steps in the Decision Process
The Issue of Protection
The Issue of Side Effects

STEPS IN THE DECISION PROCESS

Patients with uncomplicated mild hypertension, defined as DBP between 90 and 104 mm Hg, who comprise by far the largest portion of the population with an elevated blood pressure, need not immediately be started on antihypertensive drugs. Although immediate start of therapy has become common practice, a more conservative approach is recommended for the following reasons:

First, such patients are at little short-term risk and will not be endangered by postponement of drug therapy until the permanence of their hypertension is ascertained and non-drug therapies are given a chance to lower the DBP to below 90 mm Hg.

Second, many of these patients will have a persistently lower blood pressure after two to three months of repeated measurements. However, if they become normotensive, they should remain under surveillance since they are more likely to become hypertensive in the future.

Third, non-drug therapies may bring and keep their pressures down.

Fourth, and most importantly, all drug therapies have risks, costs and side effects. Though these may be minimized, they cannot be completely avoided. Often the risks of not using them clearly outweighs the risks of their use—as in patients with high overall cardiovascular risk, significant target organ damage or DBP that averages above 100 mm Hg. But many with DBP below 95 can safely be managed without drugs and many authorities, such as the Canadian Hypertension Society, advise that drugs be given only if the DBP remains above 100 mm Hg in those without target organ damage. The 1988 report of the U.S. Joint National Committee advises drug therapy for all with DBP above 95 and for higher risk patients with DBP between 90 and 94.

THE ISSUE OF PROTECTION

Despite their risks, drugs would be indicated for more patients if there were clear evidence that they protect against major cardiovascular morbidity and mortality. A number of large clinical trials completed from 1978 through 1985 have demonstrated protection against stroke (Figure 11.1, top). But protection against coronary disease, the most frequent and serious complication associated with hypertension, has not been clearly shown. In fact, higher rates of coronary mortality were noted among the treated patients in some of the trials (Figure 11.1, bottom).

The failure to demonstrate protection against coronary disease in these trials may reflect the manner by which the pressure was lowered. In most, large doses of diuretics were the first and often the only drug used. Diuretic-induced hypokalemia may have been responsible for higher rates of sudden (coronary) death.

Another reason for the failure to show protection against coronary mortality has been recognized in more recent trials of either diuretic or beta-blocker therapy: The inadvertent reduction of blood pressure to below the critical level needed to maintain myocardial perfusion, mostly in patients who have pre-existing coronary artery disease. This threshold level, in most trials, has been a diastolic blood pressure of 85 mm Hg producing a J-curve of coronary disease with blood pressures progressively lowered below that level by therapy.

Four trials have compared a diuretic against a beta-blocker to see if coronary protection could be provided by beta-blockers, which have been found to protect against recurrent myocardial infarction. In three of the four (MRC, IPPPSH, HAPPHY), the effects of the two

53

FIGURE 11.1 – A Meta-Analysis of the Effects of Antihypertensive Therapy on Mortality from Stroke and Coronary Heart Disease

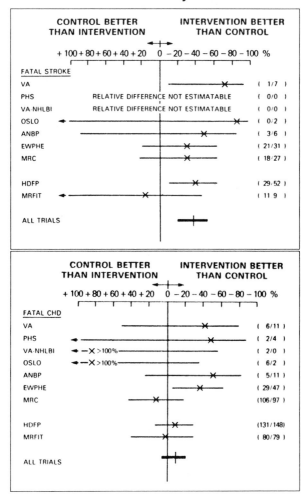

Bar graph showing estimates (X) with approximate 95 percent confidence intervals (−) of the relative difference in fatal stroke (top) and coronary heart disease (CHD) (bottom) between intervention and control groups in nine major clinical trials of the treatment of hypertension. The numbers in parentheses are the numbers of events (intervention/control). (From Cutler, et al, 1989.)

drugs were the same; in the fourth (MAPHY), the beta-blocker metoprolol provided better primary protection than a diuretic.

THE ISSUE OF SIDE EFFECTS

In most of the large clinical trials, from 20 to 40 percent of patients started on drug therapy stopped it, in about half because of adverse reactions. Even more than this percentage will have one or more side effects. Although most of these are mild and often only transient, they can and do interfere with the quality of life. Some, such as mental dullness, may be so subtle as to be inapparent to the patient (although often apparent to those around him). Others, such as impotence, may not be discussed or related to the drug (see Section #28).

The decision to start drug therapy should not be taken lightly but made with careful consideration of the implications involved. Reasonable certainty should exist that the benefits will outweigh the risks and side effects.

References

Cruickshank JM: Coronary flow reserve and the J-curve relation between diastolic blood pressure and myocardial infarction. Br Med J 1988;297:1227-1230.

Cutler JA, MacMahon SW, Furberg CD: Controlled clinical trials of drug treatment for hypertension: A review. Hypertension 1989;13(Suppl I):I-36-I-44.

IPPPSH Collaborative Group: Cardiovascular risk and risk factors in a randomized trial of treatment based on the beta-blocker oxprenolol: The international prospective primary prevention study in hypertension (IPPPSH). J Hypertens 1985; 3:379-382.

Logan AG: Report of the Canadian Hypertension Society's consensus conference on the management of mild hypertension. Can Med Assoc J 1984;131:1053-1057.

Medical Research Council Working Party: MRC trial of treatment of mild hypertension: Principle results. Br Med J 1985; 291:97-104.

Samuelsson O, et al: Cardiovascular morbidity in relation to change in blood pressure and serum cholesterol levels in treated hypertension. JAMA 1987;258:1768-1776.

Wikstrand J, et al: Primary prevention with metoprolol in patients with hypertension. JAMA 1988;259:1976-1982.

Wilhelmsen L, et al: Beta-blockers versus diuretics in hypertensive men: Main results from the HAPPHY trial. J Hypertens 1987;5:561-572.

NOTES

#12 General Guidelines for Drug Therapy

Patient Compliance

As many as half of patients who begin antihypertensive therapy will not be taking it one year later. Most of them simply stop the medication because of:

- Inadequate follow-up
- Lack of perceived benefit
- Side effects

Care must be taken to prescribe drugs in a way which:

- Can be easily remembered by asymptomatic people
- Will interfere as little as possible with various activities
- Will cause few side effects

Therapeutic Guidelines

These guidelines should help improve patient compliance to therapy:

- Establish the goal of therapy—To reduce blood pressure below 140/90 with minimal or no side effects. Use caution in achieving this goal in patients with known coronary disease to avoid the J-curve
- Educate the patient about his disease and its treatment
- Maintain contact with the patient:
  - Encourage visits and calls to allied health personnel
  - Make contact with patients who do not return
- Keep care inexpensive and simple:
  - Do the least workup needed to rule out secondary causes
  - Obtain follow-up laboratory data only yearly unless indicated more often
  - Use home blood pressure readings
  - Use non-drug, no cost therapies
  - Use the fewest daily doses of drugs needed
  - Use combination tablets when appropriate

12.

- Prescribe according to pharmacological principles:
  - Add one drug at a time
  - Start with small doses, aiming for 5 to 10 mm Hg reductions at each step
  - Prevent volume overload with adequate diuretic and sodium restriction
  - Stop unsuccessful therapy and try a different approach
  - If therapy is only partially successful, additional drugs of different classes may be added, preferably one at a time, in sufficient doses to achieve the goal of therapy
  - Anticipate side effects
  - Adjust therapy to ameliorate side effects that do not spontaneously disappear
- Be aware of the problem and be alert to signs of patient nonadherence: have the patient bring medications to the office so that pill counts and checks on numbers of refills can be done if the blood pressure has not responded

The management of resistant hypertension is discussed in Section #29.

References

Eraker SA, Kirscht JP, Becker MH: Understanding and improving patient compliance. Ann Intern Med 1984;100:258-268.

Farnett L, et al: The J-curve phenomenon and the treatment of hypertension. Is there a point beyond which pressure reduction is dangerous? JAMA 1991;265:489-495.

Greenfield S, Kaplan S, Ware JE: Expanding patient involvement in care: Effects on patient outcomes. Ann Intern Med 1985;102:520-528.

McClellan WM, et al: Continuity of care in hypertension. An important correlate of blood pressure control among aware hypertensives. Arch Intern Med 1988;148:525-528.

Zismer DK, et al: Improving hypertension control in a private medical practice. Arch Intern Med 1982;142:297-299.

#13 Diuretics: Thiazides

Usage Information
Side Effects

USAGE INFORMATION

Background

The moderately long-acting diuretic hydrochlorothiazide is the most popular drug in the United States for therapy of hypertension. Although it is now less commonly chosen as the initial drug, hydrochlorothiazide or other thiazide diuretics will almost certainly continue to be widely used. Loop diuretics and potassium-saving agents are considered in Section #14.

TABLE 13.1 — Characteristics of Diuretics

Diuretics	Daily Dosage (mg)	Duration of Action (hrs)
Thiazides		
Bendroflumethiazide (Naturetin)	1.25-2.5	More than 18
Benzthiazide (Aquatag, Exna)	12.5-50	12-18
Chlorothiazide (Diuril)	250-500	6-12
Cyclothiazide (Anhydron)	1-2	18-24
Hydrochlorothiazide (Esidrix, HydroDiuril, Oretic)	12.5-50	12-18
Hydroflumethiazide (Saluron)	12.5-50	18-24
Methyclothiazide (Enduron)	2.5-5.0	More than 24
Polythiazide (Renese)	1-4	24-48
Trichlormethiazide (Metahydrin, Naqua)	1-4	More than 24
Related sulfonamide compounds		
Chlorthalidone (Hygroton)	12.5-50	24-72
Indapamide (Lozol)	2.5	24
Metolazone (Zaroxolyn, Diulo)	1.0-5.0	24
Quinethazone (Hydromox)	50-100	18-24
Loop diuretics		
Bumetanide (Bumex)	1-10	4-6
Ethacrynic acid (Edecrin)	50-200	12
Furosemide (Lasix)	40-480	4-6
Potassium-sparing agents		
Amiloride (Midamor)	5-10	24
Spironolactone (Aldactone)	25-100	8-12
Triamterene (Dyrenium)	50-100	12

13.

Types

Thiazides are sulfonamide derivatives which cause as much as five to eight percent of the filtered sodium load to be excreted by blocking reabsorption in the early distal tubule at the cortical diluting segment. They differ in duration of action, which in turn can alter the degree of metabolic side effects. Since the mode of action and potency are similar, they share the same types of side effects.

Chemical additions to the thiazide structure provide chlorthalidone (Hygroton) with more prolonged action and indapamide (Lozol) with some additional effects on peripheral resistance and a lesser propensity to raise serum cholesterol.

Metolazone (Diulo, Zaroxolyn) also has effects within the proximal tubule so it is a more potent diuretic which will work even in the presence of significant renal insufficiency.

Mode of Action

To lower the blood pressure, diuretics must initially induce a natriuresis which shrinks blood volume. This activates various mechanisms responsible for maintenance of fluid volume, particularly the renin-angiotensin-aldosterone system. These, in turn, limit the degree of volume depletion.

At the same time, continued diuretic use leads to a fall in peripheral vascular resistance which is the major reason for the continued anti-hypertensive effect.

Most patients will achieve a 10 mm Hg fall in blood pressure with daily diuretic therapy. Those with more "volume dependent" hypertension, as demonstrable by lower levels of plasma renin activity, tend to respond particularly well. These include many black and elderly hypertensives.

Doses

Thiazides have a fairly flat dose-response curve, so that most of the antihypertensive effect is achieved with low doses (Figure 13.1). Even though as much as 200

61

FIGURE 13.1 – **Diuretic-Induced Decreases in Blood Pressure and Serum K+**

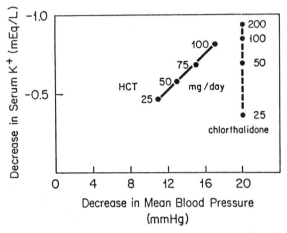

The effects of various doses of hydrochlorothiazide (HCT) and chlorthalidone on the blood pressure and serum potassium in two groups of hypertensives. The different doses of chlorthalidone and HCT were given for 6- to 8-week periods in random order. (Data on HCT taken from Degnbol, et al: Acta Med Scand 1973;193:407; data on chlorthalidone from Tweeddale, et al: Clin Pharmacol Ther 1977;22:519.)

mg of hydrochlorothiazide per day has been used in the past, as little as 12.5 mg given once a day will provide most of the blood pressure lowering effect and less of the metabolic side effects of larger doses. When added to other drugs, as little as 6.25 mg may be effective.

Despite having only a 12 to 16 hour duration of action, a single morning dose of hydrochlorothiazide will provide sustained antihypertensive effect, while reducing potassium wastage during the nighttime.

Causes for Resistance

If an inadequate response is observed with 12.5 mg of hydrochlorothiazide, the dose can be increased to 50 mg or more although little additional antihypertensive effect usually is seen above 50 mg per day. The poor response may reflect either an overwhelming load of dietary sodium or an impaired renal capacity to excrete the sodium. Patients with serum creatinine above 2.5 mg/dL likely will not respond to thiazides in usual doses.

Overly vigorous diuretic therapy may activate the renin-angiotensin-aldosterone mechanism excessively. Thereby, the antihypertensive effect of the diuretic may be antagonized by the vasoconstrictive effect of angiotensin, and potassium wastage may be increased by the aldosterone-mediated exchange of more potassium for sodium.

When more severe hypertensives are given progressively more therapy—particularly if it includes a direct vasodilator such as hydralazine—the reduction in blood pressure may lead to more intense sodium retention, mandating the use of additional diuretic. This has been noted particularly with the use of minoxidil, even more so when it is given to patients with renal insufficiency.

SIDE EFFECTS

Background

A number of side effects accompany the use of diuretics. Despite the long list of potential problems, diuretics have proven to be effective and generally safe when used in the lowest dose needed and with proper surveillance of biochemical changes.

Some side effects are allergic or idiosyncratic, such as skin rash and pancreatitis. More common are a variety of biochemical changes, which in large part reflect an exaggeration of the expected, desired effect of the drugs (Figure 13.2). Though their manifestations may not be clinically obvious, they pose more serious potential hazards during the length of time these drugs may be used.

Hypokalemia

Urine potassium wastage is inevitable with diuretic therapy. By blocking reabsorption of sodium chloride in the distal tubule, the diuretic causes additional tubular fluid containing sodium to be delivered to the lower

FIGURE 13.2—Side Effects of Diuretics

MECHANISMS BY WHICH CHRONIC DIURETIC THERAPY MAY LEAD TO VARIOUS COMPLICATIONS

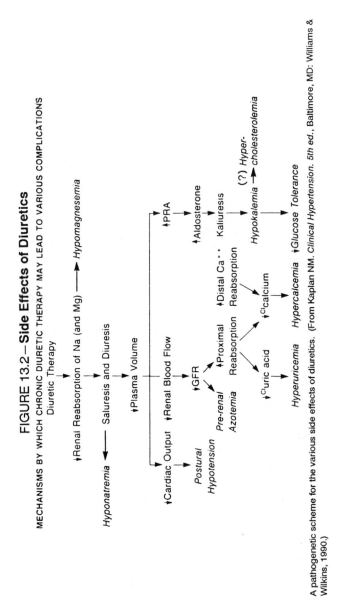

A pathogenetic scheme for the various side effects of diuretics. (From Kaplan NM. *Clinical Hypertension. 5th ed.*, Baltimore, MD: Williams & Wilkins, 1990.)

portion of the nephron wherein potassium exchange for sodium occurs. The largest amount of potassium wastage occurs initially while the diuresis is maximal, but it may continue as long as the renin-aldosterone system is activated and sodium is delivered to the collecting duct.

The average fall in plasma potassium with continuous daily diuretic therapy for four weeks or longer is 0.7 mmol/L. Depending upon the pretreatment K + level, such a fall may induce hypokalemia in approximately one-third of patients, when hypokalemia is defined as a plasma K + below 3.2 mmol/L (or serum K + below 3.5). The degree of fall in plasma K + may be greater than the fall in intracellular potassium content.

Hypokalemia rarely causes symptoms, although muscular weakness and leg cramps may be noted. However, an increase in ventricular ectopic activity has been observed and this may be responsible for the excess rates of sudden death observed in some of the large clinical trials wherein diuretic-induced hypokalemia was frequently noted and often not treated.

Hypokalemia may also be responsible for diuretic-induced glucose intolerance and hypercholesterolemia.

Diuretic-induced hypokalemia can be minimized by these steps:

- Use the smallest dose of diuretic possible
- Use moderately long-acting diuretics such as hydrochlorothiazide rather than longer-acting ones
- Reduce dietary sodium intake to 2 g (88 mmol) per day
- Increase dietary potassium intake
- Combine potassium-sparers with the diuretic (see Section #14)
- Use drugs that suppress the renin system, eg, beta-blockers, converting enzyme inhibitors

Hypercholesterolemia

As much as a 10 to 20 mg/dL increase in total serum cholesterol may develop and persist for years unless countered by reduction of saturated fat in the diet. The atherogenic potential of diuretic-induced rises in serum cholesterol has not been proven but probably is similar to "naturally" occurring hypercholesterolemia.

Glucose Intolerance and Hyperinsulinemia

Fasting and postprandial blood sugars may rise but overt hyperglycemia is rare, even in patients with pre-existing diabetes. A further rise in blood insulin levels has been noted reflecting an apparent aggravation of the peripheral insulin resistance that may accompany hypertension.

Hyperuricemia

Increased tubular reabsorption of uric acid accompanies the shrinkage of fluid volume. Diuretic-induced hyperuricemia need not be treated even if plasma levels rise above 10 mg/dL, unless gout occurs. If therapy is needed, the uricosuric agent, probenecid, is appropriate.

Hypercalcemia

More calcium is reabsorbed in a manner similar to uric acid, usually raising serum calcium levels by less than 0.5 mg/dL. Overt hypercalcemia may occur in patients with pre-existing unrecognized hyperparathyroidism.

Hyponatremia

A significant fall in plasma sodium is rarely noted, usually in elderly patients who are over-diuresed.

Hypomagnesemia

Magnesium wastage may accompany potassium wastage and hypomagnesemia occasionally develops.

References

Bennett WM, Porter GA: Efficacy and safety of metolazone in renal failure and the nephrotic syndrome. J Clin Pharmacol 1973;13:357-364.

Brand FN, et al: Hyperuricemia as a risk factor of coronary heart disease: The Framingham Study. Am J Epidemiol 1985;121:11-18.

Carlsen JE, et al: Relation between dose of bendrofluazide, antihypertensive effect, and adverse biochemical effects. Br Med J 1990;300:975-978.

Dorup I, et al: Reduced concentrations of potassium, magnesium, and sodium-potassium pumps in human skeletal muscle during treatment with diuretics. Br Med J 1988;296:455-458.

Houston MC: The effects of antihypertensive drugs on glucose intolerance in hypertensive non-diabetics and diabetics. Am Heart J 1988;115:640-656.

Jamieson MJ: Hyponatraemia. Br Med J 1985;290:1723-1728.

Kaplan NM: Our appropriate concern about hypokalemia. Am J Med 1984;77:1-4.

MacGregor GA, et al: Lack of effect of beta-blocker on flat dose response to thiazide in hypertension: Efficacy of low dose thiazide combined with beta-blocker. Br Med J 1983;286:1535-1538.

Whang R, et al: Magnesium depletion as a cause of refractory potassium repletion. Arch Intern Med 1985;145:1686-1689.

Weidmann P, Uehlinger DE, Gerber A: Antihypertensive treatment and serum lipoproteins (Editorial Review). J Hypertens 1985;3:297-306.

#14 Diuretics: Loop and K + Sparers

Loop Diuretics
Potassium-Sparing Agents

Clinical Information

Some hypertensives may require more potent diuretics than thiazides. Those who receive a thiazide may be protected from potassium wastage by the concomitant use of a potassium-sparing agent.

LOOP DIURETICS

Loop diuretics may exert a maximal natriuretic effect of 20 percent of the filtered load, some three to four times more than the thiazide diuretics, by blocking sodium chloride reabsorption in the thick ascending limb of the loop of Henle. They must enter the tubular fluid to work. Therefore, when renal blood flow is reduced, larger doses are needed. Their entry into the tubule may be competitively blocked by organic acids and drugs such as probenecid.

The two agents now available, furosemide (Lasix) and bumetanide (Bumex), are short-acting with their effect lasting three to six hours. They must be given two or three times a day to maintain the slight shrinkage of plasma volume needed to keep the blood pressure down. Therefore, they are primarily indicated for patients with reduced renal function (serum creatinine above 2.5 mg/dL) wherein thiazides are ineffectual or where there is a need for more potent diuretics as with minoxidil therapy.

Side effects are similar to those seen with thiazides with the exception of hypercalcemia. They will cause less severe biochemical changes because of shorter duration of action.

Another loop diuretic, ethacrynic acid (Edecrin) is little used because of its greater ototoxicity.

14.

POTASSIUM-SPARING AGENTS

Three potassium-sparing agents are now available, one an aldosterone antagonist, the other two inhibitors of tubular K + secretion. They are helpful in:
- Reducing thiazide-induced K + wastage
- Specifically treating hyperaldosteronism

Spironolactone (Aldactone) + HCT = Aldactazide

Spironolactone competitively blocks the uptake of aldosterone by its receptors, thereby antagonizing its actions. It will reduce diuretic-induced K + loss. However, its major use is in treatment of states of aldosterone excess, whether primary or secondary, eg, cirrhosis with ascites. Only 25 to 50 mg a day is needed for reduction in K + loss but more may be needed to block hyperaldosteronism.

Side effects include:
- Capacity to induce hyperkalemia
- Possible interference with testosterone synthesis, leading to impotence and gynecomastia in men and mastodynia in women

Triameterene (Dyrenium) + HCT = Dyazide or Maxzide

Triameterene is the K + sparer contained in combination with 25 mg of hydrochlorothiazide and sold in the United States as Dyazide. The formulation, though only 30 to 40 percent absorbed, has been widely used on a one-a-day schedule, demonstrating that as little as 10 mg of hydrochlorothiazide can provide antihypertensive effect.

Recently a better absorbed formulation of triameterene plus hydrochlorothiazide has been marketed in the U.S. as Maxzide. For most, one-half of the smaller dose containing 25 mg of HCT should be used rather than the larger dose of 50 mg.

Side effects are rare. Hyperkalemia is rarely seen except in patients with renal insufficiency who are also given potassium. Renal tubular damage and renal stones have been reported.

Amiloride (Midamor) + HCT = Moduretic

Amiloride is chemically distinct and acts differently than triameterene. However, the effects of these two K + sparers are quite similar. They both have limited natriuretic effect but inhibit K + secretion in the collecting duct. Moduretic also has 50 mg of HCT and one-half of a tablet may be adequate for most patients.

References

Andersson P-O, et al: Potassium sparing by amiloride during thiazide therapy in hypertension. Clin Pharmacol Ther 1984; 36:197-200.

Hutcheon DE, Martinez JC: A decade of development in diuretic drug therapy. J Clin Pharmacol 1986;26:567-579.

Keeton GR, Morrison S: Effects of fursemide in chronic renal failure. Nephron 1981;28:169-173.

Spence JD, Wong DG, Lindsay RM: Effects of triamterene and amiloride on urinary sediment in hypertensive patients taking hydrochlorothiazide. Lancet 1985;2:73-75.

Widmann L, Dyckner T, Wester P-O: Effects of triameterene on serum and skeletal muscle electrolytes in diuretic-treated patients. Eur J Clin Pharmacol 1988;33:577-579.

Wollam GL, et al: Diuretic potency of combined hydrochlorothiazide and furosemide therapy in patients with azotemia. Am J Med 1982;72:929-937.

#15 Adrenergic Inhibitors: Peripheral

Reserpine
Guanethidine
Guanadrel

Clinical Information

The second major class of drugs includes those which inhibit the activity of the adrenergic (sympathetic) nervous system. As shown in Table 15.1, the primary sites of action vary from the brain to the peripheral neurons. Some act as competitive inhibitors of alpha-receptors and others as blockers of beta-receptors.

The peripheral-acting agents are shown to include reserpine, which acts in the central nervous system (CNS) as well as upon peripheral neurons. These drugs are among the longest-used antihypertensives, but are now much less used as other agents have become available. Reserpine remains an effective, generally safe, inexpensive, once-a-day drug that many find works well, particularly in combination with a diuretic.

RESERPINE (Serpasil)

Reserpine, an ingredient of Indian snakeroot, acts by decreasing the transport of norepinephrine into its storage granules within the adrenergic nerve endings, thereby depleting the amount of the neurotransmitter available when the nerves are stimulated.

Small amounts are effective. When used with a diuretic, as little as 0.05 mg a day may be adequate. Larger doses of 0.25 mg are frequently used, either alone or in combination. Side effects include:

- Nasal stuffiness
- Sedation
- Mental depression

These side effects are less when using smaller doses. Patients receiving the drug should be forewarned about the symptoms of depression. Claims that reserpine use

15.

was associated with an increased risk of breast cancer have not been documented and have been attributed to bias introduced by selected exclusion of certain patients from the original studies.

GUANETHIDINE (Ismelin)

Guanethidine was a popular agent since it could be used once a day in patients with all degrees of hypertension and caused no CNS side effects. The drug caused profound inhibition of peripheral sympathetic nervous activity by blocking the exit of norepinephrine from its storage granules, frequently leading to:
- Postural hypotension
- Diarrhea
- Failure of ejaculation

Although it can be well tolerated with careful titration and avoidance of rapid postural changes, the drug has largely been relegated to a last-option status.

GUANADREL (Hylorel)

Guanadrel, a guanethidine-like agent, is easier to use because of its shorter duration of action, with less sustained interference with peripheral adrenergic action. Side effects are similar but less common. The antihypertensive efficacy is comparable to that of methyldopa.

References

Finnerty FA, Brogden RN: Guanadrel: A review of its pharmacodynamic and pharmacokinetic properties and therapeutic use in hypertension. Drugs 1985;30:22-31.

Horwitz RI, Feinstein AR: Exclusion bias and the false relationship of reserpine and breast cancer. Arch Intern Med 1985; 145:1873-1875.

TABLE 15.1 – Characteristics of Adrenergic Inhibitors

Drug	Trade Name	Dose Range (mg/day)	Side Effects
Peripheral:			
Reserpine	Serpasil	0.05-0.25	Sedation, nasal congestion, depression
Guanethidine	Ismelin	10-150	Orthostatic hypotension, diarrhea
Guanadrel	Hylorel	10-75	Orthostatic hypotension
Central:			
Methyldopa	Aldomet	500-3,000	Sedation, liver dysfunction, fever, "auto-immune" disorders
Clonidine	Catapres	0.2-1.2	Sedation, dry mouth, "withdrawal hypertension"
Guanabenz	Wytensin	8-32	Sedation, dry mouth, dizziness
Guanfacine	Tenex	1-3	Same as guanabenz
Alpha-Blocker:			
Doxazosin	Cardura	1-16	Postural hypotension, fatigue, lassitude
Prazosin	Minipress	2-20	(Same as Doxazosin)
Terazosin	Hytrin	1-20	(Same as Doxazosin)

Beta-Blockers:		
Acebutolol	Sectral	200-800
Atenolol	Tenormin	25-100
Betaxolol	Kerlone	5-20
Carteolol	Cartrol	2.5-10
Metoprolol	Lopressor	50-300
Nadolol	Corgard	40-320
Penbutolol	Levatol	10-20
Pindolol	Visken	10-60
Propranolol	Inderal	40-480
Timolol	Blocadren	20-60

Serious: bronchospasm, congestive heart failure, masking of insulin-induced hypoglycemia, depression

Less serious: poor peripheral circulation, insomnia, bradycardia, fatigue, decreased exercise tolerance, hypertriglyceridemia, decreased HDL-cholesterol

Combined Alpha- and Beta-Blocker:		
Labetalol	Normodyne, Trandate	200-1,200

Postural hypotension, beta-blocking side effects

#16 Adrenergic Inhibitors:
Central Agonists

Methyldopa
Clonidine
Guanabenz
Guanfacine

Clinical Information

Central agonists act as alpha$_2$-receptor agonists, primarily on vasomotor centers within the brain, thereby decreasing the sympathetic outflow from the CNS (Figure 16.1). As a result, cardiac output is decreased slightly but the main hemodynamic effect is a fall in peripheral vascular resistance. Although the four currently available members of this group differ in some ways, they share a common mechanism of action and side effects. Methyldopa, however, has some unique "auto-immune" side effects.

METHYLDOPA (Aldomet)

Mechanism of Action

Once the most popular drug after thiazide diuretics, methyldopa is now rarely used since beta-blockers and a steadily increasing list of newer agents have become available.

Methyldopa is converted into alpha-methylnorepinephrine which acts as an agonist (stimulant) of the central alpha-receptors. This central agonist action leads to a decrease in discharge from central vasomotor centers, dampening sympathetic nervous activity throughout the body. Blood pressure falls mainly from a decrease in peripheral resistance.

Dosage

To reduce the impact of the centrally-mediated side effects (sedation and dry mouth in particular) the initial dose should be no more than 250 mg twice a day. The total dosage can be raised to 3 g/day; however, 1 g twice

16.

FIGURE 16.1 – Mode of Action of Central Alpha$_2$-Agonists

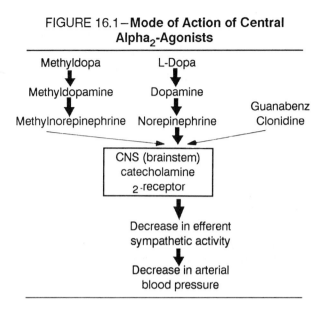

Schematic representation of the common mechanism underlying the hypotensive actions of methyldopa, clonidine and guanabenz. (From Henning M. In: van Zwieten PA (ed.) *Handbook of Hypertension*, *Vol. 3*, Amsterdam: Elsevier Science Publishers, 1984.)

a day will do almost all that is possible with the drug. One dose a day may provide 24 hour control for some, but twice a day, ie, every 12 hours, dosage is more effective for most.

Side Effects

Beyond the common sedation and dry mouth, many experience a more subtle decrease in mental alertness. These side effects are common to all four central alpha-agonists. Methyldopa, however, induces a number of "auto-immune" disorders:

- Positive Coombs tests in as many as 25 percent, but hemolytic anemia in very few
- Abnormal liver function tests in eight percent

- Severe hepatic necrosis in a small number
- Virtually every other organ has been attacked, though the frequency is quite low

These immune-inflammatory processes are not seen with the other central agonists which are equal in effectiveness. Therefore, continued use of methyldopa is difficult to justify and must be attributed to hard-to-change prescribing habits. However, patients who seem to be doing well and deny all side effects may continue to use the drug.

CLONIDINE (Catapres)

Clinical Information

Clonidine, similar to methyldopa, differs in two important ways:
- Its duration of action is shorter
- Its dosage is smaller so that it can be absorbed through the skin

Dosage

The starting dose should be 0.1 mg twice a day. The small quantity of drug needed to exert an antihypertensive effect has also been placed in a patch for transdermal absorption, thereby providing up to seven days of therapy. The patch may provide smoother control of hypertension with fewer side effects.

Side Effects

When the drug is stopped, sympathetic nervous activity may bounce back rather quickly from its suppressed state and may overshoot inducing rebound hypertension. This problem is infrequent when the total dosage is kept below 0.8 mg/day and should be treated by reinstitution of therapy.

Local skin reactions may preclude use of the transdermal patch in 20 percent or more.

GUANABENZ (Wytensin)

Clinical Information

Guanabenz is an attractive central alpha-agonist for two reasons:

- It has been shown to lower total serum cholesterol levels by five to 10 percent, unlike diuretics which tend to raise cholesterol
- It has been found to cause little reactive fluid retention, so that a diuretic may not be needed to preserve its effect

The drug mimics the mode of action and side effects of clonidine in many ways.

Dosage

Starting dosage should be 4 mg twice a day and the maximum dosage can reach a total of 64 mg/day.

Side Effects

There are few bothersome side effects beyond sedation and dryness of the mouth. This class of drugs seems particularly attractive for those who:

- Can tolerate or escape their sedative action
- Would likely not do well with beta-blockers or diuretics

These include:

- Elderly patients
- Diabetics
- Hypercholesterolemics
- Those with asthma
- Those having peripheral vascular disease

GUANFACINE (Tenex)

This agent is also similar to clonidine, although it causes less somnolence and propensity to the withdrawal syndrome.

Dosage is 1 to 3 mg once a day.

References

Byrd BF III, Collins W, Primm RK: Risk factors for severe bradycardia during oral clonidine therapy for hypertension. Arch Intern Med 1988;148:729-733.

Gehr M, MacCarthy EP, Goldberg M: Natriuretic and water diuretic effects of central alpha$_2$-adrenoceptor agonists. J Cardiovasc Pharmacol 1984;6:S781-S786.

Holmes B, et al: Guanabenz: A review of its pharmacodynamic properties and therapeutic efficacy in hypertension. Drugs 1983;26:212-229.

Kelton JG: Impaired reticuloendothelial function in patients treated with methyldopa. N Engl J Med 1985;313:596-600.

Korner PI, et al: Central and peripheral autonomic mechanisms involved in the circulatory actions of methyldopa. Hypertension 1984;6(Suppl II):II-63-70.

Schaller M-D, et al: Transdermal clonidine therapy in hypertensive patients. JAMA 1985;253:233-235.

Wilson MF, et al: Comparison of guanfacine versus clonidine for efficacy, safety and occurrence of withdrawal syndrome in step-2 treatment of mild to moderate essential hypertension. Am J Cardiol 1986;57:43E-49E.

NOTES

#17 Adrenergic Inhibitors: Alpha-Blockers

Clinical Information

Alpha$_1$-blockers currently available are doxazosin (Cardura), prazosin (Minipress) and terazosin (Hytrin).

Mode of Action

These agents have a much higher affinity for the post-synaptic alpha$_1$-receptors located on the vascular smooth muscle cells than on the presynaptic alpha$_2$-receptors located on the neuronal membrane. Blockade of the alpha$_1$-receptors inhibits the uptake of catechol-amines by the smooth muscle cells thereby blunting vasoconstriction and inducing peripheral vasodilation. Prazosin was originally thought to be a direct vasodilator but its vasodilatory action comes about via alpha$_1$-blockade (Figure 17.1).

The minimal blockade of alpha$_2$-receptors on the neuron leaves them open to the effects of catechol-amines present within the synaptic cleft. Thereby the release of additional norepinephrine (NE) from the neu-ronal storage granules is inhibited. Those non-selective alpha-blockers, phentolamine (Regitine) and phenoxy-benzamine (Dibenzyline), which also block the neuronal alpha$_2$-receptors, remove the inhibitory effect upon NE release so more NE enters the circulation, blunting the antihypertensive effect and causing tachycardia. The latter drugs are only useful for therapy of pheochro-mocytoma.

Dosage

The initial dose of an alpha-blocker may lower the blood pressure excessively, particularly in those already taking a diuretic. First-dose hypotension can be obvi-ated by:
- Stopping the diuretic for two days before
- Giving only 1 mg of the drug
- Warning the patient about the possibility of pos-tural symptoms

17.

FIGURE 17.1 – **Mode of Action of Alpha₁-Blockers**

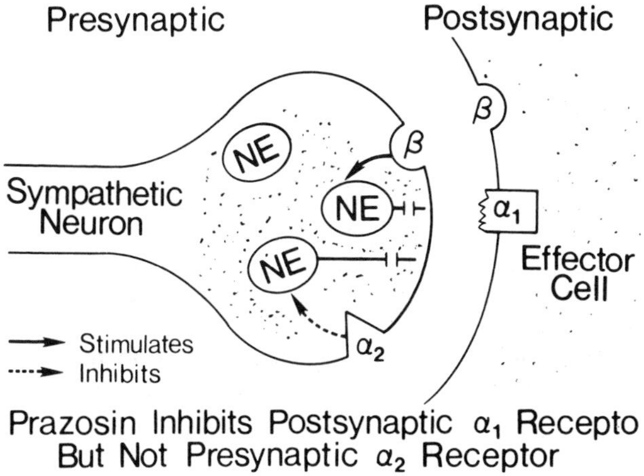

Prazosin Inhibits Postsynaptic α_1 Recepto
But Not Presynaptic α_2 Receptor

A schematic representation of a neuron and a vascular smooth muscle cell, showing how prazosin preferentially blocks the alpha₁-receptor and leaves the presynaptic alpha₂-receptor unblocked. (From Kaplan NM. *Clinical Hypertension*, 5th ed. Baltimore: Williams & Wilkins, 1990.)

Some suggest taking the first dose at bedtime. To preclude trouble if the patient arises from bed during the night, the first dose may be taken on a day when the patient can lie around and better manage postural symptoms. In fact, the problem is very infrequent particularly with the slower acting doxazosin and terazosin.

Dosage should be slowly increased up to a maximum of 20 mg a day. Prazosin should be taken twice a day, whereas doxazosin and terazosin can be given once daily.

Side Effects

Beyond the very rare first-dose hypotension, some patients continue to experience dizziness and a few others GI distress. Alpha-blockers rarely cause CNS side effects such as sedation or dry mouth.

Lipid and Metabolic Effects

Beta-blockers often raise serum triglycerides and lower HDL-cholesterol levels (see Section #19). Alpha-blockers appear to do the opposite:

- Total cholesterol and triglyceride levels are lowered
- HDL-cholesterol is raised in many patients

Selective alpha$_1$-receptor blockers are particularly useful in young patients who wish to remain physically active. In such patients, the use of beta-blockers often reduces exercise capacity by lowering cardiac output. This class of drugs provides good antihypertensive effects without worsening lipids or lowering potassium, as do diuretics.

Moreover, prazosin has been shown to reduce plasma insulin levels and improve glucose tolerance.

References

Frishman WH, Eisen G, Lapsker J: Terazosin: A new long-acting alpha$_1$-adrenergic antagonist for hypertension. Med Clin N Amer 1988;72:441-448.

Pollare T, et al: Application of prazosin is associated with an increase of insulin sensitivity in obese patients with hypertension. Diabetologia 1988;31:415-420.

Pool JL: Effects of doxazosin on serum lipids: A review of the clinical data and molecular basis for altered lipid metabolism. Am Heart J 1991;121:251-260.

Talseth T, Westlie L, Daae L: Doxazosin and atenolol as monotherapy in mild and moderate hypertension: A randomized, parallel study with a three-year follow-up. Am Heart J 1991; 121:280-285.

Van Zwieten PA, Timmermans PBMWM, Van Brummelen P: Role of alpha-adrenoceptors in hypertension and in antihypertensive drug treatment. Am J Med 1984;77:17-25.

Walker RG, et al: Prazosin: Long-term treatment of moderate and severe hypertension and lack of "tolerance." Med J Aust 1981;2:146-147.

#18 Adrenergic Inhibitors: Beta-Blockers, Part I

Clinical Information

Beta-blockers have become the second most widely used drugs after diuretics. They provide numerous benefits, but their adverse effects on lipids and glucose-insulin need to be considered. Those which have partial agonist or intrinsic sympathomimetic activity (ISA) may provide all of the benefits with fewer adverse effects.

Mode of Action

Beta-blockers with no ISA (Figure 18.1) lower the blood pressure by:
- Reducing cardiac output
- Inhibiting the release of renin
- Reducing norepinephrine release from neurons
- Decreasing central vasomotor activity

In the peripheral vessels, beta-blockade inhibits vasodilation. Therefore, unopposed alpha-mediated vasoconstriction increases peripheral vascular resistance. This limits the antihypertensive effect and is responsible for the side effect of cold extremities.

Beta-blockers with ISA, eg, pindolol, acebutolol and penbutolol lower the blood pressure without reducing cardiac output and may decrease peripheral resistance by causing some sympathetic stimulation while blocking endogenous catechol effects. They cause less bradycardia and cold extremities.

Differences Among Beta-Blockers

Beyond different degrees of ISA, beta-blockers differ in lipid solubility and relative selectivity in blocking $beta_1$-receptors in the heart versus $beta_2$-receptors elsewhere.

The more lipid soluble, the more of the drug that is taken up and metabolized on the first pass through the liver and the more of the drug that enters the brain. The greater hepatic uptake results in inactivation of the first few doses until uptake is saturated. A small IV dose may produce much greater effects than a larger oral dose.

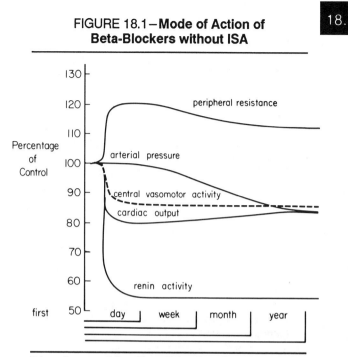

18

FIGURE 18.1 – **Mode of Action of Beta-Blockers without ISA**

Schematic representation of the multiple actions of beta-blocker therapy over variable periods of time. The solid lines have been measured; the dotted line of central vasomotor activity has not been measured. (Adapted from Birkenhager WH, et al. Therapeutic effects of beta-adrenoceptor blocking agents in hypertension. In: Frick P, et al. *Advances in Internal Medicine and Pediatrics, No. 39.* Berlin: Springer-Verlag, 1977:117-134.)

Lipid soluble agents generally have shorter duration of action because of more rapid hepatic inactivation. However, in the relatively large doses used to treat hypertension, most beta-blockers will provide 24-hour antihypertensive effects with one dose a day.

Comparable lipid solubility is:
- Very soluble:
  - Propranolol
  - Metoprolol
  - Timolol
  - Penbutolol

89

- Intermediate solubility:
  - Pindolol
  - Acebutolol
  - Betaxolol
- Less soluble:
  - Atenolol
  - Nadolol
  - Carteolol

Those which are less lipid soluble remain unmetabolized in the blood and are slowly excreted through the kidneys; therefore, their duration of action is longer. Less enters the brain, and there seem to be fewer CNS side effects.

Beta-blockers which are more active on cardiac $beta_1$-receptors than on $beta_2$-receptors include:

- Acebutolol
- Atenolol
- Betaxolol
- Metoprolol

This selectivity can be shown with acute administration of single doses. These agents cause less decrease in peripheral blood flow or pulmonary air movement than noncardioselective agents. However, none are truly cardioselective, and most differences disappear with chronic use or larger doses.

Clinical Effectiveness

The antihypertensive effectiveness of the various beta-blockers in equivalent doses is similar.

When used alone, beta-blockers appear to be more effective in patients who are younger and white and less effective in elderly and black patients. This difference may reflect lower plasma renin levels in elderly and black patients.

Beta-blockers may be particularly useful in patients with:

- Hypertension associated with tachycardia and high cardiac output
- Hypertension accompanied by:
  - Angina
  - Migraine

- Glaucoma
- Other coincidental diseases which are responsive to beta-blockade

Beta-blockers have been shown to reduce recurrent myocardial infarction and sudden death among patients who recently experienced an acute MI. However, as noted in Section #11 (*The Decision to Use Drugs*), in only one of four large trials have beta-blockers been found to reduce the incidence of initial MIs below that seen with diuretic-based therapy. In that trial (MAPHY), the beta-blocker was metoprolol.

References

Boissel J-P, et al: Secondary prevention after high-risk acute myocardial infarction with low-dose acebutolol. Am J Cardiol 1990;66:251-260.

Frishman WH: Clinical perspective on celiprolol: Cardioprotective potential. Am Heart J 1991;121:724-729.

Frishman WH, et al: Betaxolol: A new long-acting $beta_1$-selective adrenergic blocker. J Clin Pharmacol 1990;30:686-692.

Man in't Veld AJ, Van den Meiracker AH, Schalekamp MA: Do beta-blockers really increase peripheral vascular resistance? Review of the literature and new observations under basal conditions. Am J Hypertens 1988;1:91-96.

van Baak MA, Struyker Boudier HAJ, Smits JFM: Antihypertensive mechanisms of beta-adrenoceptor blockade: A review. Clin Exper Hypertension 1985;A7:1-72.

van der Meiracker AH, et al: Acute and long-term effects of acebutolol on systemic and renal hemodynamics, body fluid volumes, catecholamines, active renin, aldosterone, and lymphocyte beta-adrenoceptor density. J Cardiovasc Pharmacol 1988;11:413-423.

Wikstrand J, et al: Primary prevention with metoprolol in patients with hypertension. JAMA 1988;259:1976-1982.

#19 Adrenergic Inhibitors: Beta-Blockers, Part II

Side Effects
Overview of Therapy

Clinical Information

Beta-blockers may be associated with various side effects. Most are predictable in view of their pharmacological action. Some side effects are more common in those which are noncardioselective or lipid soluble or which lack intrinsic sympathomimetic activity (ISA).

SIDE EFFECTS

Cardiac

Beta-blockers with little or no ISA induce bradycardia, which may be asymptomatic and should be disregarded. Those who monitor the degree of physical activity by heart rate should be made aware that maximal heart rate will be approximately 20 percent lower. The state of physical conditioning can be achieved in the presence of beta-blockade, but reduced exercise ability and easier fatigue are often noted, less so with ISA beta-blockers.

Beta-blockers tend to slow the rate of A-V conduction and may worsen the degree of heart block. The decrease in cardiac output with non-ISA beta-blockers may push a few patients who are near decompensation already into congestive heart failure.

Pulmonary

Bronchospasm may result if patients are in need of beta-agonist effects to maintain patent airways. Cardioselective beta-blockers may decrease air movement. However, if beta-agonist bronchodilators are required, they will be more effective in the presence of a more cardioselective beta-blocker.

Metabolic

Diabetics who take insulin and are prone to hypoglycemia should be given beta-blockers with great caution. The response to hypoglycemia largely depends upon catecholamine stimulation of glucose synthesis and release, particularly in insulin-dependent diabetics who are also unable to secrete glucagon. Insulin-induced hypoglycemia may be longer in duration and more severe in the presence of a beta-blocker. The beta-blockers mask the usual symptoms of hypoglycemia such as:

- Tremor
- Tachycardia
- Hunger

Sweating, however, is not diminished, and diabetics given beta-blockers should be aware of the significance of sweating as a warning signal.

Hypertriglyceridemia and a concomitant fall in HDL-cholesterol are common with beta-blockers, though less marked or not at all with those having high degrees of ISA. Serum triglyceride levels rise an average of 30 percent with most beta-blockers (Figure 19.1). These lipid abnormalities may be responsible for the failure of beta-blocker therapy to reduce the incidence of coronary heart disease in controlled therapeutic trials.

The insulin resistance and hyperinsulinemia present in hypertension may be further aggravated by beta-blockers.

Central

Fatigue is common. It may be related to the decreased cardiac output seen with non-ISA beta-blockers or to central effects. Bad dreams, even hallucinations, may be noted. Depression has been said to be more common with the use of propranolol. These effects are less common with the lipid-insoluble agents and in those with ISA.

FIGURE 19.1 — **Effects of Beta-blockers on Lipids**

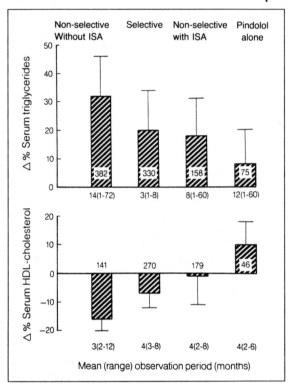

Mean percentage responses of serum triglycerides and HDL-cholesterol to monotherapy with different types of beta-blockers (mean ± s.d.). ISA - intrinsic sympathomimetic activity. Numbers in columns denote the total numbers of reported cases used for analysis. (From Weidman P, et al. J Hypertension 1985;3:297.)

Renal

A 10- to 20-percent fall in renal blood flow and glomerular filtration rate has been noted with most beta-blockers, though not with nadolol. The effect may reflect renal vasoconstriction.

Fluid retention has been noted in a small number of low-renin hypertensives given propranolol.

OVERVIEW OF THERAPY

In the past 15 years, beta-blockers have been increasingly used as first or second drug in the treatment of hypertension. They are effective and usually well tolerated. However, they may cause fatigue and loss of exercise ability that many patients may not relate to the drug. Of more concern are the lipid and glucose-insulin abnormalities seen with those which lack ISA.

These drugs protect against recurrent MIs but have not been shown in most studies to protect against the first heart attack. The multiple side effects preclude their use in as many as 25 percent of patients. If a beta-blocker is chosen for the treatment of hypertension, one with ISA would seem to be the best choice since it will probably cause fewer side effects which are clinically obvious and biochemically important.

References

Avorn J, Everitt DE, Weiss S: Increased antidepressant use in patients prescribed beta-blockers. JAMA 1986;255:357-360.

Bauer JH: Adrenergic blocking agents and the kidney. J Clin Hypertens 1985;3:199-221.

Dornhorst A, Powell SH, Pensky J: Aggravation by propranolol of hyperglycaemic effect of hydrochlorothiazide in type II diabetics without alteration of insulin secretion. Lancet 1985; 1:123-126.

Frcka G, Lader M: Psychotropic effects of repeated doses of enalapril, propranolol, and atenolol in normal subjects. Br J Clin Pharmacol 1988;25:67-73.

Herbertsson P, Fagher B: Effects of verapamil and atenolol on exercise tolerance in 5,000 m cross-country running: A double-blind cross-over study in normal humans. J Cardiovasc Pharmacol 1990;16:23-27.

Pollare T, et al: Metabolic effects of diltiazem and atenolol: Results from a randomized, double-blind study with parallel groups. J Hypertension 1989;7:551-559.

Weidmann P, Uehlinger DE, Gerber A: Antihypertensive treatment and serum lipoproteins (Editorial Review). J Hypertens 1985;3:297-306.

#20 Adrenergic Inhibitors: Combined Alpha- and Beta-Blockers

Clinical Information

Labetalol (Normodyne, Trandate) is the only drug currently available which has both alpha- and beta-blocking effects within the same structure (Figure 20.1). It is available for both oral and intravenous use.

Mode of Action

In smaller doses, the drug has three times more beta-blocking effect than alpha-blocking action. A maximal degree of alpha-blockade occurs with increasing doses, whereas the beta-blocking effects continue so that the ratio increases to 6:1 or higher.

The beta-blocking action is similar to that seen with propranolol, which is noncardioselective and lipid soluble. The alpha-blocking effect is similar to that seen with prazosin, inducing peripheral vasodilation. As a result of the combination of effects, blood pressure falls mainly from a decrease in peripheral resistance with little effect on heart rate or cardiac output. Little change is noted in renin or catechol levels and renal function is not altered.

When taken by mouth, its lipid solubility results in extensive first pass hepatic metabolism so that only about 25 percent is bioavailable. The duration of action is eight to 12 hours.

When given intravenously, the antihypertensive effect is rapid and may be profound, with a propensity to postural hypotension if the patient stands.

Dosage

By mouth, 100 mg twice a day is usually an adequate starting dose with a maximum of 2,400 mg per day. By vein, the drug may be given initially in a 20 mg dose by slow injection, with repeated 20 to 80 mg doses at 10 minute intervals. The maximal effect of each dose is usually seen within 10 minutes, and the duration of action

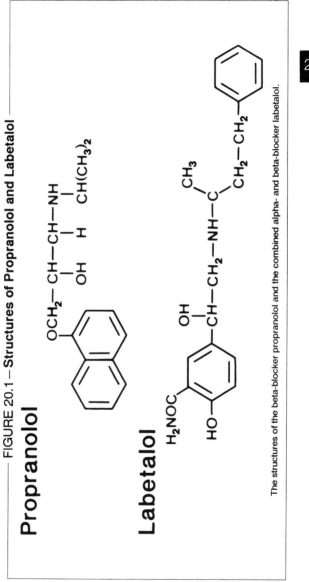

— FIGURE 20.1 — Structures of Propranolol and Labetalol

The structures of the beta-blocker propranolol and the combined alpha- and beta-blocker labetalol.

97

is up to six hours. The drug may also be given by slow continuous infusion at an initial rate of 2 mg per minute, with 50 to 200 mg usually required for an adequate response.

Side Effects

Some side effects are related to alpha-blockade:
- Postural dizziness
- Scalp tingling
- Nasal stuffiness

Other side effects are related to beta-blockade:
- Fatigue
- Vivid dreams
- Bronchospasm
- Cold extremities
- Claudication

In addition, the drug may cause GI distress with:
- Nausea
- Vomiting
- Pain
- Diarrhea
- Constipation

Clinical Use

Orally, labetalol should be used primarily for treatment of moderate to severe degrees of hypertension. Intravenously, it should be useful in those who have a need for rapid, though not instantaneous, reduction of markedly elevated blood pressure. Those who do not require nitroprusside but who need parenteral therapy can be given labetalol rather than diazoxide or hydralazine. This may be an advantage in being able to quickly switch the patient to chronic oral therapy with the same drug.

References

DeQuattro V, et al: Labetalol blunts morning pressor surge in systolic hypertension. Hypertension 1988;11(Suppl I):I-198-201.

Feit A, et al: Effect of labetalol on exercise tolerance and double product in mild to moderate essential hypertension. Am J Med 1985;78:937-941.

Lebel M, et al: Labetalol infusion in hypertensive emergencies. Clin Pharmacol Ther 1985;37:615-618.

Prichard BNC: Combined alpha- and beta-receptor inhibition in the treatment of hypertension. Drugs 1984;28(Suppl 2):51-68.

Szlachcic J, et al: Left ventricular hypertrophy reversal with labetalol and propranolol: A prospective, randomized, double-blind study. Cardiovasc Drugs Ther 1990;4:427-434.

#21 Vasodilators: Direct-Acting

Clinical Information

Two vasodilators, hydralazine and minoxidil, directly dilate arterioles. Others whose effects are similar but whose modes of action are different include the angiotensin-converting enzyme inhibitors and the calcium entry blockers (see Sections #22 and #23 and Table 21.1).

The use of direct-acting vasodilators has been made practical by combining them with diuretics and adrenergic inhibitors (Figure 21.1). Ser-Ap-Es is such a combination of small amounts of hydralazine with hydrochlorothiazide and reserpine. In more recent years, larger doses of hydralazine and minoxidil have been used as part of triple therapy to treat severe degrees of hypertension.

These drugs alone induce significant dilation of resistance arterioles with a fall in peripheral resistance. The resultant fall in blood pressure activates baroreceptors which set off sympathetic reflexes, causing:

- Release of both renin and catecholamines
- Stimulation of the heart
- Constriction of veins

The fall in blood pressure also leads to renal retention of sodium, expanding fluid volume.

Various side effects (Figure 21.1) are seen as a result of all of these compensatory reactions to the vasodilator-induced fall in blood pressure, including:

- Tachycardia
- Flushing
- Headaches
- A loss of antihypertensive efficacy

With the concomitant use of an adrenergic inhibitor and a diuretic, the various compensatory reactions are inhibited and the blood pressure falls even more, thus reducing side effects. A beta-blocker may be used as the adrenergic inhibitor. However, others, such as clonidine or guanfacine, may also be used. A thiazide is usually

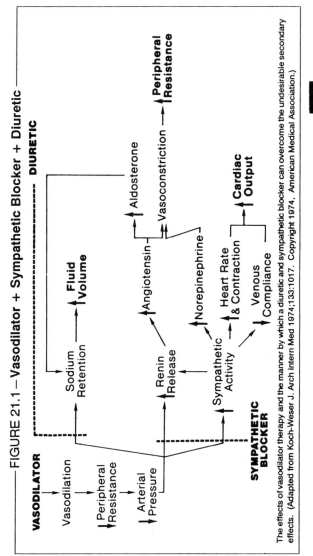

— FIGURE 21.1 — Vasodilator + Sympathetic Blocker + Diuretic —

The effects of vasodilator therapy and the manner by which a diuretic and sympathetic blocker can overcome the undesirable secondary effects. (Adapted from Koch-Weser J. Arch Intern Med 1974;133:1017. Copyright 1974, American Medical Association.)

chosen as the diuretic, but furosemide or metolazone may be needed in those who have a marked response to minoxidil, particularly if they start with some degree of renal insufficiency.

Clinical Use

Hydralazine has often been chosen as the third drug for those not responding adequately to a diuretic and an adrenergic inhibitor. The initial dose is usually 25 mg twice a day and may be increased to 200 mg twice a day, although total daily doses beyond 200 mg are associated with an increasing likelihood of a lupus-like reaction.

Minoxidil is often used for patients with severe hypertension, particularly when renal insufficiency is present. It can be given once a day with total dosage from 5 to 60 mg. Its use is complicated by a marked tendency for:

- Fluid retention—Requiring use of potent diuretics
- Hirsutism—Precluding use of the drug in many women unwilling to have hair on their face and elsewhere

Men are rarely concerned, and the drug is now available for use as a topical treatment to regrow hair on bald heads.

Side Effects

Most side effects are attributable to the activation of compensatory mechanisms to direct vasodilation, including:

- Tachycardia
- Flushing
- Headache

However, hydralazine also can cause a lupus-like reaction with:

- Fever
- Rash
- Arthralgias

Renal or CNS involvement is rare. The reaction is usually benign and disappears when the drug is stopped. Perry, et al, found that patients who have a reaction have no residual damage and a 10- to 15-year longer survival rate than similar patients who have not had a reaction.

The tendency for fluid retention and hirsutism with minoxidil reflects its marked vasodilation of renal and skin arterioles.

Overview

Vasodilators are effective and generally well tolerated. However, their use has been receding in the face of equally effective ACE inhibitors and calcium entry blockers which tend to cause fewer side effects.

TABLE 21.1 – Characteristics of Approved Vasodilators

Drug	Trade Name	Dose Range (mg/day)	Side Effects
Direct Vasodilators			
Hydralazine	Apresoline	50-400	Headaches, tachycardia (if used alone), lupus-like syndrome
Minoxidil	Loniten	5-100	Headaches, fluid retention, hirsutism
Calcium Entry Blockers			
Diltiazem	Cardizem	120-240	Nausea, headache, conduction defects
Isradipine	Dynacirc	5-40	Flush, headache, local ankle edema
Nicardipine	Cardene	30-90	(same as Isradipine)
Nifedipine	Procardia	20-120	(same as Isradipine)
Verapamil	Calan, Isoptin, Verelan	240-480	Constipation, headache, conduction defects
Angiotensin-Converting Enzyme Inhibitors			
Benazepril	Lotensin	10-40	Cough, loss of taste, skin rash
Captopril	Capoten	25-150	Rare: Leukopenia, proteinuria, angioneurotic edema
Enalapril	Vasotec	5-20	
Fosinopril	Monopril	10-40	
Lisinopril	Prinivil, Zestril	10-60	
Quinapril	Accupril	10-40	
Ramipril	Altace	1.25-10	

References

Eggertsen R, Hansson L: Vasodilators in hypertension: A review with special emphasis on the combined use of vasodilators and beta-adrenoceptor blockers. Int J Clin Pharmacol Ther Toxicol 1985;23:411-423.

Mansilla-Tinoco R, et al: Hydralazine, antinuclear antibodies, and the lupus syndrome. Br Med J 1982;284:936-939.

Oh MS, et al: Minoxidil in a once-a-day step-3 antihypertensive program. J Clin Hypertens 1985;1:23-29.

Perry HM Jr, et al: Survival in hydralazine-treated hypertensive patients with and without late toxicity. J Chron Dis 1977;30:519-528.

Silas JH, Ramsay LE, Freestone S: Hydralazine once daily in hypertension. Br Med J 1982;284:1602-1604.

Taverner D, et al: Improvement of renal function during long-term treatment of severe hypertension with minoxidil. Quart J Med 1983;206:280-287.

#22 Vasodilators: Calcium
Entry Blockers

Clinical Information
The calcium entry blockers (CEBs) now available include:

- Diltiazem (Cardizem)
- Isradipine (Dynacirc)
- Nicardipine (Cardene)
- Nifedipine (Procardia)
- Verapamil (Calan, Isoptin, Verelan)

Nicardipine and isradipine are "second generation" CEBs and offer even greater vasoselectivity than the others. A number of other CEBs, most of which are dihydropyridines similar to nicardipine and nifedipine, are under investigation. These agents are among the fastest growing drugs, having been added to the choices for initial monotherapy in the 1988 JNC-4 report.

Mode of Action
All calcium antagonists lower the blood pressure by reducing calcium entry into vascular smooth muscle cells. The decrease in free intracellular calcium reduces vascular tone and contractility. Peripheral resistance and blood pressure fall.

Diltiazem and verapamil also act within the S-A and A-V nodes, making them useful for the treatment of certain arrhythmias but adding to their interaction with beta-blockers to induce serious A-V conduction block. Dihydropyridines such as nicardipine and nifedipine have no effect upon sinus or A-V nodal conduction. This is an advantage in reducing beta-blocker interactions and a disadvantage in allowing for some reflex tachycardia.

Clinical Use
Most of these are available in the U.S. in fairly short-acting formulations requiring three doses per day for a sustained 24-hour antihypertensive effect. Verapamil and diltiazem are available in a sustained-release form for twice-a-day therapy, isradipine is used twice-a-day

and nifedipine is available in a slow-release tablet which allows once-a-day therapy. These drugs have been found by some to work better in older patients than in younger patients and particularly well in blacks.

Considerable experience with liquid nifedipine, given either sublingually or swallowed, has shown that it lowers blood pressure markedly within 20 minutes.

Although calcium blockers have not been previously noted to protect patients after an acute myocardial infarction, such protection has been shown in a large trial (DAVIT II) with verapamil.

22.

Side Effects

The nature and severity of side effects differ considerably among the drugs, reflecting different effects at various sites such as peripheral vasodilation (dihydropyridines > verapamil > diltiazem) and A-V conduction (verapamil > diltiazem, dihydropyridines none at all). The most common side effects with each include:

- Diltiazem:
  - Nausea
  - Ankle edema
  - Headache
  - Rash
- Nicardipine, nifedipine and isradipine:
  - Flushing
  - Headache
  - Postural dizziness
  - Nausea
  - Ankle edema
- Verapamil:
  - Constipation
  - Postural dizziness
  - Headache
  - Nausea

The edema seen with dihydropyridines is not generalized and is localized to the ankles or legs, likely secondary to vasodilation. It may be so cosmetically bothersome as to preclude the use of these drugs, particularly nifedipine.

Verapamil is most likely to cause:
- Myocardial depression
- Excessive bradycardia
- A-V nodal dysfunction

It should rarely be used with beta-blockers.

Although the secretion of most hormones is dependent upon local release of calcium, hormonal secretions are affected very little by these drugs and they may be safely used in diabetics.

Overview

Calcium entry blockers are effective antihypertensives. They will continue to be widely used with the availability of more vasoselective and longer-acting preparations. The potential to protect against both cardiac and vascular damage, as shown experimentally and in one large trial of post-MI patients, and the ability to reduce the blood pressure particularly well in elderly patients, as shown in a few clinical trials, have led to widespread use of calcium entry blockers as antihypertensive agents.

References

Brouwer RML, Follath F, Buhler FR: Review of the cardiovascular adversity of the calcium antagonist beta-blocker combination: Implications for antihypertensive therapy. J Cardiovasc Pharmacol 1985;7(Suppl 4):S38-S44.

Burris JE, et al: An assessment of diltiazem and hydrochlorothiazide in hypertension. Application of factorial trial design to a multicenter clinical trial of combination therapy. JAMA 1990;263:1507-1512.

Cummings DM, et al: The role of calcium channel blockers in the treatment of essential hypertension. Arch Intern Med 1991;151:250-259.

Danish Study Group on Verapamil in Myocardial Infarction: Effect of verapamil on mortality and major events after acute myocardial infarction (The Danish Verapamil Infarction Trial II—DAVIT II). Am J Cardiol 1990;66:779-785.

Henry PD: Atherosclerosis, calcium, and calcium antagonists. Circulation 1985;72:456-459.

Kaplan NM: Calcium entry blockers in the treatment of hypertension: Current status and future prospects. JAMA 1989;262:817-823.

Man in't Veld AJ: The place of isradipine in the treatment of hypertension. Am J Hypertens 1991;4:96S-102S.

M'Buyamba-Kabangu JR, et al: Relative potency of a beta-blocking and a calcium entry blocking agent as antihypertensive drugs in black patients. Eur J Clin Pharmacol 1986;29:523-527.

Meredith PA, et al: Age and the antihypertensive efficacy of verapamil: An integrated pharmacodynamic-pharmacokinetic approach. J Hyperten 1987;5(Suppl 5):S219-S221.

Opie LH: Calcium channel antagonists, Part III: Use and comparative efficacy in hypertension and supraventricular arrhythmias. Minor indication. Cardiovasc Drug Ther 1988;1:625-656.

Pollare T, et al: Metabolic effects of diltiazem and atenolol: Results from a randomized, double-blind study with parallel groups. J Hypertension 1989;7:551-559.

#23 Vasodilators: Angiotensin-Converting Enzyme Inhibitors

Clinical Information

Multiple ACE inhibitors are now available, and a larger number are under clinical investigation (Table 23.1). As a group, they provide excellent antihypertensive action with few bothersome side effects. Initial experiences with captopril when used in large doses for therapy of resistant hypertension reported a high frequency of side effects. The frequency and severity of side effects have fallen progressively as these drugs have been given in smaller doses to patients with milder hypertension and good renal function. ACE inhibitors are now approved for use for all degrees of hypertension and are of particular value when congestive heart failure coexists.

TABLE 23.1 — New and Investigational ACE Inhibitors According to the Ligand of the Zinc Ion

Sulfhydryl-Containing Inhibitors
- Alacepril
- Altiopril
- Zofenopril

Carbozyl-Containing Inhibitors
- Benazepril
- Cilazapril
- Delapril
- Perindopril
- Quinapril
- Ramipril
- Spirapril

Phosphoryl-Containing Inhibitors
- Fosinopril
- SQ 29852

Mode of Action

The conversion of the inactive prohormone angiotensin I (A-I) to the potent vasoconstrictor angiotensin II (A-II) is accomplished by an ACE available throughout the body. By ingenious molecular manipulation, biochemists engineered a drug which competitively inhibited the converting enzyme by attaching to its binding sites on the A-I structure. The ACE inhibitors block completely the synthesis of A-II so that all of the effects of the hormone are countered. A-II mediated vasoconstriction is overcome and the blood pressure falls. A-II mediated synthesis of aldosterone is inhibited, thereby sodium retention and potassium wastage are reduced (Figure 23.1).

23

FIGURE 23.1 – **Mode of Action of ACE Inhibitors**

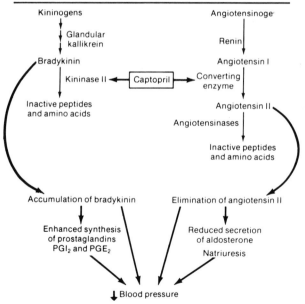

The mechanisms by which captopril and other converting enzyme inhibitors may lower the blood pressure. (From Kaplan NM, *Clinical Hypertension*, 5th ed. Baltimore: Williams & Wilkins, 1990.)

ACE is the same enzyme which inactivates the vasodepressor hormone bradykinin. Inhibition of this inactivation may allow the vasodepressor effect to persist, so this effect may be involved in the antihypertensive action of the drug. High levels of bradykinin may be responsible for the cough seen with these drugs. In addition, captopril (but not enalapril) appears to directly stimulate the synthesis of vasodilatory prostaglandins in renal and vascular endothelium.

Peripheral resistance and the blood pressure fall as a result of these effects. Cardiac output does not increase, possibly because of inhibition of the expected baroreceptor-mediated reflex increase in sympathetic activity as a result of the absence of A-II. Despite marked falls in blood pressure, heart rate rarely rises.

The ability to reduce systemic vascular resistance without cardiac stimulation make ACE inhibitors particularly useful as unloading agents in the treatment of congestive heart failure wherein high levels of A-II are usually found.

Clinical Use

Smaller doses of ACE inhibitors are being used to treat milder degrees of hypertension, eg:
- Captopril 12.5 to 25 mg twice a day
- Enalapril 5 to 10 mg twice a day
- Lisinopril 10 to 20 mg once a day
- Fosinopril 10 to 20 mg once a day

Small doses should be used as initial therapy in those suspected of high renin-angiotensin forms of hypertension since they may experience a precipitous first-dose hypotension when the support of the blood pressure by A-II is acutely removed. In particular, patients with bilateral renovascular hypertension, wherein high levels of A-II have served to maintain renal blood flow beyond the stenoses, may experience a marked fall in blood pressure and loss of renal function with ACE inhibitor therapy. Patients with unilateral renovascular hypertension tend to respond well to the drug, and it is the usual choice for medical therapy.

112

Side Effects

Side effects may be related to:
- Pharmacological effect of the drug:
  - Cough
  - Hypotension
  - Loss of renal function
- The sulfhydryl group contained within captopril, but not in enalapril or lisinopril, may be responsible for more, such as:
  - Rash
  - Loss of taste
  - Glomerulopathy with proteinuria
  - Leukopenia

The latter symptoms seem to be less common with enalapril or lisinopril but the difference may reflect the wider exposure of patients to high doses of captopril.

Overview

These agents are being widely used in the treatment of milder degrees of hypertension as well as the more severe, resistant forms. They work particularly well in those with higher renin levels, including those on diuretics. Research in animals shows the agents may protect against renal damage better than other drugs that lower the blood pressure as well. Research in patients with high-to-normal renin levels suggest that they may correct an underlying fault of tissue responses to A-II. The outlook seems particularly promising. Moreover, the availability of additional agents with different ligands of the zinc ion of ACE (see Table 21.1) provides additional potential benefits. For example, fosinopril has a balanced route of elimination which shifts toward the liver in the presence of renal impairment. Therefore, this agent may prove particularly useful in elderly hypertensives who often have some degree of renal insufficiency.

References

Bucknall CE, et al: Bronchial hyperreactivity in patients who cough after receiving angiotensin converting enzyme inhibitors. Br Med J 1988;296:86-88.

Croog SH, et al: The effects of antihypertensive therapy on the quality of life. N Engl J Med 1986;314:1657-1664.

Guntzel P, et al: The effect of cilazapril, a new angiotensin converting enzyme inhibitor, on peak and trough blood pressure measurements in hypertensive patients. J Cardiovasc Pharmacol 1991;17:8-12.

Gupta RK, et al: Platelet function during antihypertensive treatment with quinapril, a novel angiotensin-converting enzyme inhibitor. J Cardiovasc Pharmacol 1991;17:13-19.

Heber ME, et al: First dose response and 24-hour antihypertensive efficacy of the new once-daily angiotensin-converting enzyme inhibitor, ramipril: Am J Cardiol 1988;62:239-245.

Penner SB, et al: Long-term captopril in young and old patients with mild hypertension. J Clin Pharmacol 1991;31:65-71.

Pollare T, Lithell H, Berne C: A comparison of the effects of hydrochlorothiazide and captopril on glucose and lipid metabolism in patients with hypertension. N Engl J Med 1989;321:868-873.

Salvetti A: Newer ACE inhibitors. A look at the future. Drugs 1990;40:800-828.

Schofield PM, et al: Which vasodilator drug in patients with chronic heart failure? A randomized comparison of captopril and hydralazine. Br J Clin Pharmac 1991;31:25-32.

Sullivan PA, et al: Fosinopril, an angiotensin-converting enzyme inhibitor, and propranolol: Comparative effects at rest and exercise on blood pressure, hormonal variables, and plasma potassium in essential hypertension. Cardiovasc Drugs Ther 1989;3:57-62.

van Schaik BAM, et al: Pharmacokinetics of lisinopril in hypertensive patients with normal and impaired renal function. Eur J Clin Pharmacol 1988;34:61-65.

Williams GH, Hollenberg NK: Are non-modulating patients with essential hypertension a distinct sub-group? Am J Med 1985; 79(Suppl 3C):3-9.

#24 Step-Care vs. Individualized Substitution

Step-Care

In the past, most American practitioners used the step-care approach to therapy: Start with one drug and add a second, a third, and a fourth in sequence if the response is inadequate. For most, the first step has been a thiazide diuretic, and this group of drugs has become the most widely prescribed in North America. Elsewhere, diuretics are less commonly chosen as first drug.

The diuretic-first, step-care approach was recommended in the 1977 and 1980 reports of the U.S. Joint National Committee (JNC), a group of hypertension experts appointed by the head of the National Heart, Lung, and Blood Institute to formulate guidelines for the detection, evaluation and treatment of hypertension. The 1984 report of the Third JNC and the Canadian Hypertension Society broadened the choice of first drug to either a diuretic or a beta-blocker.

In the 1988 report of the JNC, the traditional approach was broadened to include four classes of drugs as choices for initial therapy: diuretics, beta-blockers, ACE inhibitors and calcium entry blockers. The author believes that alpha-blockers and central alpha-agonists may also be appropriate.

Beyond the broadening of choices for initial therapy, the report recommended individualizing therapy on the basis of the following special considerations:

- Demographic features
- Concomitant disease and therapies
- Lifestyle
- Physiologic and biochemical measurements
- Economic considerations

More about factors to be considered in the choice of initial therapy (after or along with non-drug therapies) will be covered below under *Substitution* approach. The overall approach to therapy that seems most appropriate is shown in Figure 24.1.

FIGURE 24.1 – **Individualized Therapy**

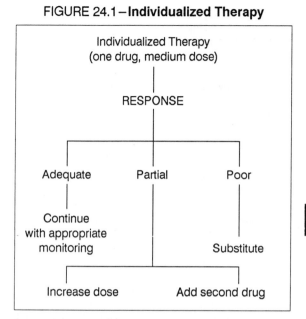

An appropriate framework for therapy of the majority of patients with uncomplicated, fairly mild hypertension.

Substitution

In addition to broadening the choice of first drug, consideration should be given to a different approach than the step-wise addition of a second drug if the first proves inadequate. Although it is true that all antihypertensive drugs approved for use have similar efficacy for the overall hypertensive population, there are differences in responses to different drugs among certain groups of patients and among individual patients.

For example, younger and white patients generally respond better to an adrenergic inhibitor or an angiotensin-converting enzyme inhibitor. Older and black patients may respond better to a diuretic or a calcium antagonist. These differences may reflect differences in plasma renin activity or the differing contributions of various pathogenic mechanisms.

Beyond these general differences, individual patients of the same type may respond variably to any one drug. What works well for one elderly black female may do little for another. Rather than immediately adding another drug as second step, the wiser course is to stop the first drug which has proven ineffectual and try one from another class of drugs. The number of drugs will be minimized and effectiveness will be maximized.

The step-care approach seems more appropriate for patients with significant hypertension, wherein the first drug provides a definite effect but not enough to bring the considerably elevated pressure to the goal of therapy. Although any given dose of antihypertensive agent will apparently be more effective the higher the initial blood pressure, it should be noted that most drugs have a limited efficacy. The addition of a second or third drug is indicated if a partial but definite effect has been achieved with the first drug.

Eighty percent of all hypertensives are in the mild category, ie, DBP between 90 and 104 mm Hg. Half of these have DBP between 90 and 95 mm Hg (Figure 2.1). For these, one drug may be enough to accomplish a 5 to 10 mm Hg fall in DBP. If the first drug does not accomplish the goal, another should be substituted rather than added.

References

Kaplan NM: Maximally reducing cardiovascular risk in the treatment of hypertension. Ann Intern Med 1988;109:36-40.

Laragh JH: Lessons from antihypertensive drug trials that employed "stepped care:" The case for rationalized individualized treatment strategies based on renin system patterns. J Cardiovasc Pharmacol 1984;6:S1067-S1072.

Muller FB, et al: Calcium antagonists and the second drug for hypertensive therapy. Am Med J 1986;81(Suppl 6A):25-29.

Reid JL: Hypertension 1988: Present challenges and future strategies. J Hypertens 1988;6:3-8.

#25 The Choice of First Drug

Clinical Information

A large number of drugs can be chosen for initial therapy. The choice should be made carefully. If the patient responds well, the drug may be taken for many years; therefore, inapparent biochemical and other side effects must be avoided. If the patient does not respond well or has significant side effects with the first drug, he may be dissuaded from returning for follow-up care.

The majority of patients have mild hypertension which should be adequately managed with one drug. In most of the therapeutic trials involving patients with DBP from 90 to 109 mm Hg, 40 to 60 percent of patients had pressure brought to below 90 (and often had at least a 10 mm Hg absolute fall) with one drug. Therefore, the choice of the first drug is an important one.

Past Choices

A thiazide diuretic has been the usual first choice in the U.S. more than elsewhere. However, a number of concerns have risen about their use, particularly in the high doses often prescribed:

- In various therapeutic trials wherein diuretics were the first (and often the only) drug, protection against coronary disease has not been uniformly seen. In half of these trials, more coronary mortality, mostly due to sudden death, was seen among the treated patients (see Section #11, Figure 11.1)
- Diuretic-induced hypokalemia has sometimes been shown to invoke ventricular ectopic activity, suggesting this as a mechanism for the increase in sudden deaths in the trials
- The 10 to 20 mg/dL rise in serum cholesterol and the further resistance to insulin seen with diuretics may counter the long-term protection against coronary disease provided by the lowered blood pressure

Present Choices

Rather than using a set formula for all patients, various features of each patient should be considered in making the most appropriate choice, one that will more likely lower the blood pressure to the desired level and leave the patient unencumbered by bothersome side effects. The three major features that should prove most helpful are demographics, lifestyle and concomitant diseases (Table 25.1).

Some advocate that therapy be based upon various biochemical measurements, such as plasma renin activity or hemodynamic functions. The author does not believe these are needed. Although the cost of therapy ought not to enter into the decision, those who cannot afford more expensive drugs may have to take less expensive ones even if they are not the preferred choices. Fortunately, with the increasing availability of once-a-day formulations, fewer tablets should be needed so that the daily cost of therapy should be kept minimal.

25

TABLE 25.1 – Individualized Approach to Initial Therapy

PATIENT CHARACTERISTICS	PREFERRED DRUGS	LESS PREFERRED DRUGS
Demographic Features		
Age below 50	Alpha-blocker Beta-blocker ACE inhibitor	Diuretic
Age over 65	Thiazide diuretic Calcium entry blocker ACE inhibitor	Central alpha-agonist
Black race	Thiazide diuretic	Beta-blocker ACE inhibitor
White race	Beta-blocker ACE inhibitor	
Life-Style		
Physically active	Alpha-blocker ACE inhibitor Calcium entry blocker	Beta-blocker
Need to avoid sedation	All other	Central alpha-agonist
Noncompliant	Once-a-day dosage	Central alpha-agonist

TABLE 25.1 continued ➡

TABLE 25.1 – Individualized Approach to Initial Therapy (continued)

PATIENT CHARACTERISTIC	PREFERRED DRUGS	LESS PREFERRED DRUGS
Concomitant Diseases		
Coronary heart disease	Beta-blocker Calcium entry blocker	Direct vasodilator
Post-myocardial infarction	Beta-blocker	
Congestive heart failure	ACE inhibitor Direct vasodilator Thiazide diuretic	Beta-blocker Calcium entry blocker
Supraventricular tachyarrhythmias	Verapamil Beta-blocker	
Bradycardia, sick sinus		Beta-blocker Diltiazem, verapamil
Cerebrovascular disease		Central alpha-agonist
Hypercholesterolemia	Alpha-blocker ACE inhibitor Calcium entry blocker	Diuretic Beta-blocker
Hypertriglyceridemia	Alpha-blocker	Beta-blocker (non-ISA)
Migraine	Beta-blocker	
History of depression		Central alpha-agonist Reserpine Beta-blocker
Peripheral vascular disease	ACE inhibitor Calcium entry blocker Alpha-blocker	Beta-blocker
Renal insufficiency	Loop diuretic Minoxidil ACE inhibitor	Thiazide diuretic K+ -sparing agent
Collagen disease	ACE inhibitor Calcium entry blocker	Methyldopa Hydralazine
Diabetes mellitus	ACE inhibitor Central alpha-agonist Alpha-blocker	Thiazide diuretic Beta-blocker
Gout		Diuretic
Asthma		Beta-blocker
Osteoporosis	Diuretic	

References

Beevers DG, et al: Comparison of lisinopril versus atenolol for mild to moderate essential hypertension. Am J Cardiol 1991; 67:59-62.

Black HR: Metabolic considerations in the choice of therapy for the patients with hypertension. Am Heart J 1991;121:707-715.

Freis ED: Age and antihypertensive drugs (hydrochlorothiazide, bendroflumethiazide, nadolol, and captopril). Am J Cardiol 1988;61:117-121.

Kaplan NM: Therapy of mild hypertension: An overview. Am J Cardiol 1984;6:S833-S836.

Laragh JH: Modification of stepped care approach to antihypertensive therapy. Am J Med 1984;77:78-86.

Saunders E, et al: A comparison of the efficacy and safety of a beta-blocker, a calcium channel blocker, and a converting enzyme inhibitor in hypertensive blacks. Arch Intern Med 1990;150:1707-1713.

Schwartz GL: Initial therapy for hypertension—individualizing care. Mayo Clin Proc 1990;65:73-87.

#26 The Choice of Second Drug

Clinical Information

Whatever agent other than a diuretic is chosen as first drug, a diuretic will often be chosen as second. The addition of a diuretic will increase the antihypertensive efficacy of other types of drugs. This reflects not only the expected antihypertensive effect derived from the action of the diuretic, but also the ability of the diuretic to remove excess fluid that may have been retained by the kidneys of hypertensive patients when blood pressure is reduced. In addition to overcoming this "side effect" of non-diuretic therapy, the combination may blunt some of the side effects of the diuretic. If the initial choice has been either a beta-blocker or an ACE inhibitor, the hypokalemia often induced by the diuretic may be prevented presumably because these drugs block the diuretic-induced rises in renin-aldosterone. No information is available as to whether the prevention of potassium wastage will also prevent the hypercholesterolemic effect of diuretics.

Small vs. Large Doses

Before further consideration of the individual choices and combinations, a more general question needs attention: Should maximal doses of the first drug be used before a second, or should smaller doses of two (or even more) drugs be used? Arguments can be made for either course.

In favor of maximal doses of the first are these: Patients are more likely to take one medication, and most medications come in single, larger-dose tablets. If partial success is achieved with a smaller dose, more success is likely with a large dose. If the patient has had no problem with the initial dose, little trouble should be seen with increasing dosage.

In favor of smaller doses of two (or more) drugs are these: Most antihypertensive drugs have a fairly flat dose-response curve. Most of the antihypertensive effect of hydrochlorothiazide is achieved with 25 mg a day, and raising the dose to 50 or even 100 mg provides relatively little additional antihypertensive effect. Side effects are often dose-related. Fifty or 100 mg of HCT will cause increasingly more potassium wastage (Figure 13.1). Appropriate combinations of smaller doses of two antihypertensive agents (usually a diuretic plus another) are available, and no more tablets or doses need to be taken.

There is no certain right answer. The step-care approach was predicated, in part, upon the concept that addition of second or third drugs in smaller doses was preferable to larger doses of single agents.

Available Choices

Although diuretics will generally be added as second drug if a non-diuretic is the first, numerous other rational combinations are available if there are reasons to avoid a diuretic (Table 26.1).

Few will tolerate effective doses of a direct vasodilator (hydralazine or minoxidil) in the absence of an adrenergic inhibitor to blunt the reflex sympathetic activity that usually accompanies the lowering of blood pressure by vasodilation. Neither ACE inhibitors nor calcium entry blockers tend to activate baroreceptors as much as do the direct vasodilators, though they act as vasodilators. Baroreceptor reactivity tends to become blunted with patients' advancing age. Elderly patients may tolerate direct vasodilators when given alone or with a diuretic.

Two Drugs Without a Diuretic

If the initial dose is an adrenergic inhibitor, the second need not be a diuretic, particularly in patients with circumstances where the biochemical side effects of diuretics need to be avoided such as:
- Gout
- Diabetes
- Irritable hearts

26

TABLE 26.1 – Rational Combinations of Antihypertensive Agents

FIRST CHOICE	SECOND CHOICE
Adrenergic inhibitor	ACE inhibitor Calcium entry blocker Diuretic Other type of adrenergic inhibitor
ACE inhibitor	Adrenergic inhibitor Calcium entry blocker Diuretic
Calcium entry blocker	ACE inhibitor Adrenergic inhibitor Diuretic
Diuretic	ACE inhibitor Adrenergic inhibitor Calcium entry blocker

The choice could be another adrenergic inhibitor that acts in a different manner or a vasodilator. There is no reason to add a second drug that works in the same manner as the first, such as clonidine plus methyldopa or two beta-blockers.

The addition of a vasodilator as second drug when the initial drug is an adrenergic inhibitor may be more logical. The one exception would be if an alpha-blocker is the first drug, since its effect, though mediated by alpha-blockade, is as a vasodilator. Though more vasodilation may be achieved by adding another vasodilator that acts in a different manner, the better choice would likely be one from another class of drug.

References

Joint National Committee on Detection, Evaluation, and Treatment of High Blood Pressure: The 1988 report of the Joint National Committee on Detection, Evaluation, and Treatment of High Blood Pressure. Arch Intern Med 1988;148:1038.

Muller FB, et al: Calcium antagonists and the second drug for hypertensive therapy. Am J Med 1986;81(Suppl 6A):25-29.

van Schaik BAM, et al: Comparison of enalapril and propranolol in essential hypertension. Eur J Clin Pharmacol 1986; 29:511-516.

Weinberger MH: Blood pressure and metabolic responses to hydrochlorothiazide, captopril, and the combination in black and white mild-to-moderate hypertensive patients. J Cardiovasc Pharmacol 1985;7:S52-S55.

#27 The Choice of Third Drug

Clinical Information

Perhaps 10 percent of hypertensive patients will require more than two drugs to achieve adequate control of the blood pressure. The same arguments for and against adding three drugs in smaller doses rather than taking two drugs to their highest doses can be made, with the exception of being able to provide all three in one tablet. The only single tablet containing three drugs in the U.S. and Canada is Ser-Ap-Es. The dose of both reserpine and hydrochlorothiazide would be excessive with more than three tablets a day as would be required to provide adequate control of significantly high blood pressure.

Logical Combinations

Most use one of each of the following major categories when triple therapy is needed:
- Diuretic
- Adrenergic inhibitor
- Vasodilator

Hydralazine has been the most popular vasodilator, with minoxidil reserved for those with renal insufficiency. Increasingly, either an ACE inhibitor or a calcium entry blocker is being chosen instead. An alpha-blocker may be used as the vasodilator component of triple therapy since it acts in that manner.

Even for patients with severe hypertension, once-a-day dosage with minoxidil, a beta-blocker and a diuretic can be effective, as noted by Spitalewitz, et al.

Making a Choice

Which of these various combinations is best? There are no properly conducted clinical trials to provide the answer. One study, by McAreavey, et al, compared five different drugs (hydralazine, labetalol, methyldopa, minoxidil, and prazosin) and a placebo in 240 patients whose DBP remained above 95 mm Hg on a full dose of diuretic and a beta-blocker. The six choices were allocated in a random manner, each to about 40 of the patients. Those given the combined alpha/beta-blocker labetalol had their beta-blocker stopped, and only men were given minoxidil. The protocol precluded any change in the dose of diuretic or beta-blocker, with the third drug added in progressively larger doses to a predetermined maximum. Each patient was treated for six months, and the effects on blood pressure, as well as the number of patients able to continue on each drug, were determined.

As seen in Figure 27.1, minoxidil was clearly the most effective drug. But the design of the trial, which precluded increases in diuretic therapy, caused all but 10 of the minoxidil-treated patients to stop the drug because of fluid retention. The other four drugs were equal in their antihypertensive effects, all superior to placebo. However, fewer than half given labetalol or methyldopa were able to continue them for six months. Three-fourths of those given either hydralazine or prazosin were able to complete the trial.

This trial is the only one of its kind and was begun before either ACE inhibitors or calcium blockers were available. In view of the difficulty in doing such controlled studies, it is unlikely that more will be done. The choice of third drug will have to continue to be made on logical assumptions as to which is better. Calcium entry blockers and ACE inhibitors will increasingly be chosen.

Need for More Diuretic

The results with minoxidil indicate the frequent need for additional diuretic, often potent loop diuretics, to overcome the marked renal fluid retention that may follow successful reduction of the blood pressure with the potent vasodilator. Similar, though less striking, fluid retention may accompany the use of other drugs. Doses of diuretic that may have seemed adequate initially may no longer be enough. Despite all of the prior warnings about excessive diuretic therapy, there may be a need to give more to patients whose response to other drugs seems to be inadequate or fading.

FIGURE 27.1 – The Study by McAreavey, et al

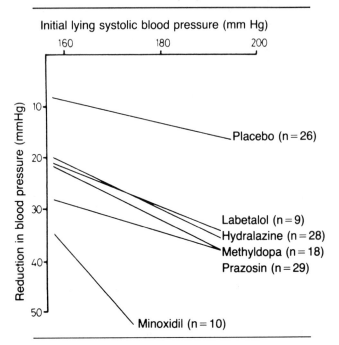

Regression lines relating reduction in blood pressure to initial lying
systolic pressure for each drug group in randomized trial of placebo and
five drugs in patients whose DBP remained > 95 on diuretic and beta-
blocker. N in parentheses refers to number of patients in each group who
were able to complete the study. (From McAreavey D, Ramsey LE,
Lathem, et al. Br Med J 1984;288:106.)

References

Guazzi MD, et al: Calcium-channel blockade with nifedipine and angiotensin-converting-enzyme inhibition with captopril in the therapy of patients with severe primary hypertension. Circulation 1984;70:279-284.

McAreavey D, et al: "Third drug" trial: Comparative study of antihypertensive agents added to treatment when blood pressure remains uncontrolled by a beta-blocker plus thiazide diuretic. Br Med J 1984;288:106-111.

Opie LH, Jennings AA: Role of calcium channel blockade in chronic hypertension following successful management of hypertensive emergency. Am Med J 1986;81 (Suppl 6A):35-42.

Potter JF, Beevers DG: Comparison of nifedipine and captopril as third-line agents in hypertensive patients uncontrolled with beta-blocker and diuretic therapy. J Clin Pharmacol 1987;27: 410-414.

Spitalewitz S, Porush JG, Reiser IW: Minoxidil, nadolol, and a diuretic. Arch Intern Med 1986;146:882-886.

#28 Step-Down Therapy and Side Effects

Step-Down Therapy
Impotence

STEP-DOWN THERAPY

Clinical Information

Just as a minority of patients may be resistant to therapy, a large percentage of patients may be so sensitive as to be able to reduce the level of medication. In carefully-controlled follow-up studies, about 15 percent of patients whose hypertension was well-controlled on medications for five years have remained normotensive for up to five years after therapy was completely discontinued. In a study of a group of such patients who were enrolled in the Hypertension Detection and Follow-up Program, the percentage whose pressures remain down is greater if they lose weight or reduce dietary sodium intake.

Causes

It is unknown why some patients who have not lost weight, reduced sodium intake, etc. are able to stop therapy, assuming they were truly hypertensive when therapy was started. The argument can be made that since only 15 percent will remain normotensive off therapy, successful therapy should not be stopped, particularly because of the potential hazard of recurrence and progression of hypertension if the patient does not remain under observation. A larger group of patients whose pressures become normotensive on therapy may be able to reduce the level of therapy, ie, step-down, rather than stop therapy altogether.

This may occur because the patient is following one or more of the non-drug therapies described in Sections #9 and #10 or because the underlying mechanisms responsible for the development of hypertension have become quiescent or have been reversed by the lowering of pressure for some time. Structural hypertrophy of resistance vessels may regress.

All who have been normotensive for a year or longer should attempt to reduce the dosage of medication. If more than one medication is being taken, only one should be reduced at a time. In one study, the dose of diuretic could be halved in most patients without a loss of blood pressure control but with a reduction in diuretic-induced hypokalemia.

IMPOTENCE

Clinical Information

Of various side effects of therapy (Table 28.1), inability to gain and maintain an erection is perhaps the least well understood and managed. Most of the individual side effects are related to the mode of action of the various drugs. Loss of erectile potency may accompany the use of any antihypertensive agent. In the first two years of the MRC trial, impotence was noted in 10 percent of men on placebo, 13 percent on a beta-blocker, and 23 percent on thiazide diuretic.

This surprisingly higher frequency with diuretic therapy may reflect the greater blood pressure lowering effect initially observed with diuretics in the MRC trial. Hypertensive men may have considerable atherosclerotic narrowing of the arteries bringing blood into the penis. Penile blood flow may diminish further if the head of pressure within this area of the circulation is reduced significantly by effective antihypertensive therapy more so than elsewhere. Since erection requires a 10-fold increase in blood flow, the occurrence of impotence can be looked upon as a non-specific effect of successful lowering of the blood pressure.

Causes

Certain drugs, particularly central alpha agonists, may cause more impotence by interfering with neurogenic control of penile function. Impotence may be purely psychogenic reflecting the concerns of middle-aged men who suddenly find themselves to have hypertension, but many become impotent because their pressures are brought down too much and too fast. In common with cerebral blood flow, too great and sudden a fall in blood pressure may cause tissue hypoperfusion. Therefore, the lowering of blood pressure should be gradual and gentle. If impotence appears with any one drug, the patient should discontinue use of the drug and be watched to see if potency returns. If it does, another type of drug should be used. The switch of therapy can be made if the pressure is so high as not to allow discontinuation of therapy, with encouragement that the switch may make a difference.

Loss of sexual desire or libido is rarely an organic problem caused by antihypertensive medications and is more likely psychogenic in origin. A drug such as spironolactone which can interfere with testosterone synthesis may cause loss of libido.

References

Alderman MH, et al: Antihypertensive drug therapy withdrawal in a general population. Arch Intern Med 1986; 146:1309-1311.

Bancroft J, Wu FC: Erectile impotence. Br Med J 1985;290: 1566-1568.

Finnerty FA Jr: Stepped-down therapy versus intermittent therapy in systemic hypertension. Am J Cardiol 1990;66:1373-1374.

Grimm RH, et al: Beneficial effects from systematic dosage reduction of the diuretic, chlorthalidone: A randomized study within a clinical trial. Am Heart J 1985;109:858-864.

Langford HG, et al: Dietary therapy slows the return of hypertension after stopping prolonged medication. JAMA 1985; 253:657-664.

Nelson RP: Nonoperative management of impotence. J Urol 1988;139:2-5.

Schmieder RE, Rockstroh JK: When is discontinuation of antihypertensive therapy indicated? Cardiovasc Drugs Ther 1990;4:1487-1494.

Virag R, Bouilly P, Frydman D: Is impotence an arterial disorder? Lancet 1985;1:181-184.

TABLE 28.1 ➡

TABLE 28.1 – Side Effects of Antihypertensive Drugs

Drugs	Side Effects	Precautions and Special Considerations
Thiazides and related Sulfonamide Compounds	Hypokalemia, hyperuricemia, glucose intolerance, hypercholesterolemia	May be ineffective in renal failure; hypokalemia increases digitalis toxicity; hyperuricemia may precipitate acute gout; may increase blood levels of lithium
Loop diuretics	Same as for thiazides	Hyponatremia, especially in the elderly
Potassium-sparing agents	Hyperkalemia	Danger of hyperkalemia in patients with renal failure
Amiloride Spironolactone	Gynecomastia, mastodynia	
Triamterene	Renal calculi	

Peripheral-acting adrenergic inhibitors		
Guanadrel	Orthostatic hypotension and diarrhea	Use cautiously in elderly patients because of orthostatic hypotension
Guanethidine	Same as for guanadrel	Same as for guanadrel
Rauwolfia alkaloids, reserpine	Lethargy, nasal congestion	Contraindicated with history of mental depression; use with caution with history of peptic ulcer
Central-acting adrenergic inhibitors		
Clonidine	Drowsiness, dry mouth, fatigue	Rebound hypertension may occur after abrupt discontinuance
Guanabenz	Same as for clonidine	
Guanfacine	Same as for clonidine	
Methyldopa	Same as for clonidine	May cause liver damage, positive direct Coombs' test, other auto-immune disorders
Alpha$_1$-Adrenergic blocker		
Doxazosin	Orthostatic hypotension, weakness and palpitations	Delete diuretics to minimize orthostatic hypotension
Prazosin		
Terazosin		

(continued) ⇒

TABLE 28.1 — Side Effects of Antihypertensive Drugs (continued)

Drugs	Side Effects	Precautions and Special Considerations
Beta-Adrenergic blockers (Less in those with ISA)	Bradycardia, fatigue, insomnia, bizarre dreams, hypertriglyceridemia, decreased HDL cholesterol; depression	Should not be used in patients with asthma, chronic obstructive pulmonary disease, congestive failure, heart block (greater than first degree), and sick sinus syndrome; use with caution in patients with diabetes and peripheral vascular disease
Combined alpha- and beta adrenergic blockers		
Labetalol	Asthma, nausea, fatigue, dizziness and headache	Same contraindications as with beta-blockers
Vasodilators	Headache, tachycardia, and fluid retention	May precipitate angina in patients with coronary heart disease
Hydralazine	Positive antinuclear antibody	Lupus syndrome may occur
Minoxidil	Hypertrichosis, fluid retention	May cause or aggravate pleural and pericardial effusions

Angiotensin-converting enzyme inhibitors Benazepril Captopril Enalapril Fosinopril Lisinopril Quinapril Ramipril	Rash, loss of taste, cough, hyperkalemia, hypotension	Can cause reversible, acute renal failure in patients with bilateral renal arterial stenosis; neutropenia may occur in patients with autoimmune-collagen disorders; proteinuria may worsen but usually improves
Calcium-entry blockers		
Diltiazem	Headache, flushing, and dizziness	Use with caution in patients with congestive failure or heart block
Isradipine	Nausea	
Nicardipine	Flushing, local edema	
Nifedipine	Flushing, local edema	
Verapamil	Flushing, local edema	
	Constipation	Same as for diltiazem

#29 Resistant Hypertension

Volume Overload

Some patients may not respond to appropriate antihypertensive therapy because of reactive fluid retention (see Section #27). Of the multiple reasons for resistance to therapy (Table 29.1), volume overload due either to inadequate diuretic therapy or to excessive sodium intake is the most common problem.

The problem may not become obvious until the blood pressure is partially lowered. This creates an even greater tendency for sodium retention by the hypertensive patient's kidneys, which have been reset to tolerate a higher head of pressure without excreting extra volume. When the pressure is lowered, even to levels well within the normal range, the hypertensive patient's kidneys may respond by retaining more sodium and water in a misguided attempt to bring the pressure back to the higher level to which they have adjusted.

Therefore, blood pressures that have been successfully lowered may begin to gradually increase, a process called "pseudo-tolerance" since it is caused by reactive fluid retention and not by a true tolerance or tachyphylaxis to the antihypertensive therapy. Doses of diuretic that were adequate may need to be increased. Amounts of dietary sodium that did not appear to be excessive may need to be reduced.

The problem is most common with those antihypertensive agents that stimulate the renin-aldosterone mechanism, such as direct-acting vasodilators (hydralazine or minoxidil) and less common with those that suppress it, such as beta-blockers and ACE inhibitors. Calcium entry blockers may actually be natriuretic and, therefore, less likely to cause fluid retention.

Inadequate Dosages or Drug Interference

In addition to the need for supplementary or more potent diuretics, the doses of other antihypertensives may need to be increased either because inadequate amounts have been prescribed or because their effects are being antagonized. The doses may be too low

TABLE 29.1 – Causes of Refractory Hypertension

Nonadherence to therapy

Drug related
- Doses too low
- Inappropriate combinations (eg, two centrally acting adrenergic inhibitors)
- Rapid inactivation (eg, hydralazine)
- Effects of other drugs
  - Sympathomimetics
  - Antidepressants
  - Adrenal steroids
  - Nonsteroidal anti-inflammatory drugs
  - Nasal decongestants
  - Oral contraceptives

Associated conditions
- Increasing obesity
- Alcohol intake more than one ounce of ethanol a day
- Renal insufficiency
- Renovascular hypertension
- Malignant or accelerated hypertension
- Other causes of hypertension

Volume overload
- Inadequate diuretic therapy
- Excessive sodium intake
- Fluid retention from reduction of blood pressure
- Progressive renal damage

29.

because some patients inactivate the drugs more rapidly. The acetylation of hydralazine is genetically determined to be slow or rapid; hepatic blood flow and metabolism may be increased by other drugs, food or nicotine.

A number of other drugs may antagonize the effects of antihypertensive agents. Some of them do so by stimulating the sympathetic nervous system, eg, phenylpropanolamine in diet pills and nasal decongestants, amphetamine and cocaine. Others, such as antidepressants, block the action of drugs that work via neuronal uptake, eg, guanethidine and methyldopa. Nonsteroidal anti-inflammatory drugs decrease the effects of diuretics, beta-blockers and ACE inhibitors, perhaps by decreasing levels of vasodilatory prostaglandins.

Associated Conditions

Other conditions that may elevate the blood pressure may either have been present all along and missed or have developed after therapy was begun. The importance of the pressor effect of alcohol intake greater than two ounces a day is described in Section #9. Renal damage from progressive nephrosclerosis is particularly common in blacks, whereas diabetics are susceptible to progressive glomerular sclerosis. As renal function deteriorates, hypertension often worsens, likely from sodium retention.

Renovascular Hypertension

Of all the secondary forms of hypertension, renovascular disease is the most common among those with resistant hypertension. As noted in Section #5, it is particularly common among those with rapidly progressive disease and was found in one-third of a series of 123 patients with accelerated or malignant hypertension.

Overview

The cause of resistant hypertension should be recognizable. It may take hospitalization but that step should only rarely be necessary and, in fact, may be misleading. The blood pressure almost always falls in the hospital but may rise again after discharge, even without obvious changes in therapy.

If the cause can be identified, relief may be simple. If not, larger doses of more potent drugs may be required.

References

Gifford RW, Tarazi RC: Resistant hypertension: Diagnosis and management. Ann Intern Med 1978;88:661-665.

Ramsay LD, Silas JH, Freestone S: Diuretic treatment of resistant hypertension. Br Med J 1980;281:1101-1103.

Singer DRJ, et al: Captopril and nifedipine in combination for moderate to severe essential hypertension. Hypertension 1987;9:629-633.

Swales JD, et al: Treatment of refractory hypertension. Lancet 1982;1:894-896.

Toner JM, Close CF, Ramsay LE: Factors related to treatment resistance in hypertension. Q J Med 1990;77:1195-1204.

Webster J: Interactions of NSAIDs with diuretics and beta-blockers: Mechanisms and clinical implications. Drugs 1985;30:32-41.

Winickoff RN, Murphy PK: The persistent problem of poor blood pressure control. Arch Intern Med 1987;147:1393-1396.

#30 Special Patients: Children, the Elderly and Blacks

Hypertension in Children
Hypertension in the Elderly
Hypertension in Blacks

HYPERTENSION IN CHILDREN

Clinical Information

Hypertension in prepubertal children is:
- Rare
- Often symptomatic
- Usually secondary

Hypertension in postpubertal children and adolescents is:
- More common
- Usually asymptomatic
- More likely primary (or idiopathic)

Since blood pressures have been taken more frequently among young people, the presence of hypertension in as many as one percent of seemingly healthy adolescents has been recognized.

Different criteria for hypertension in children of various ages have been proposed in the JNC 4 report. These are the suggested upper limits of normal BP in children by age, from JNC 4:

Age/Years	Blood Pressure
3 to 5	< 116/76
6 to 9	< 122/78
10 to 12	< 126/82
13 to 15	< 136/86

Prepubertal

The younger the patient with elevated blood pressure, the more likely it represents a congenital problem.

These include:
- Coarctation of the aorta
- Renal hypoplasia
- Congenital adrenal hyperplasia

Most advise a study of renal function and structure for every prepubertal child with hypertension without an obvious cause, involving one of the following:
- An IVP (most common in the past)
- Ultrasound
- Digital subtraction arteriography

Postpubertal

The older the child, the more likely hypertension is primary. Obesity is a major factor, and weight reduction should be the first approach to therapy. Guidelines as to when to institute drug therapy and which drug should be used remain unsettled.

Some believe that evidence of left ventricular hypertrophy by echocardiography, present in a surprisingly high percentage of adolescents with presumably mild hypertension, is an indication for the use of drug therapy. More information is needed since some LVH may be a necessary response to the elevated afterload from increased vascular resistance.

HYPERTENSION IN THE ELDERLY

Clinical Information

As many as half of people over age 65 will develop systolic hypertension, defined as a BP above 160 mm Hg. People who develop significant diastolic hypertension after age 60 should be evaluated for renovascular disease. Isolated systolic hypertension reflects increasing atherosclerotic rigidity of large arteries. Some who have very high cuff blood pressure readings may have "pseudo-hypertension" from inability of the balloon to compress the calcified brachial artery. Such falsely high readings should be suspected if the radial artery remains palpable after the Korotkoff sounds disappear (Osler's sign).

30.

The presence of isolated systolic levels above 160 mm Hg is associated with an increased risk of stroke and other cardiovascular disease (CVD). However, data have not been available as to the ability of antihypertensive therapy to lower such pressures or to remove the risks of CVD. A placebo-controlled study, Systolic Hypertension in the Elderly Program, has been reported and indicates that therapy is beneficial.

Therapy

Elderly people free of target organ damage with diastolic levels above 95 mm Hg should be treated since they are protected as well, if not better, than young patients by appropriate therapy. Non-drug therapy (see Sections #9 and #10) should be tried since elderly people may have more problems with drugs due to various age-related changes, including:

- Loss of baroreceptor responsiveness, increasing their propensity to postural hypotension
- Decrease in myocardial contractility
- Shrinkage of body fluid volume
- Decrease in renal excretory capacity
- Inability to remember doses and to open child-resistant bottles of drugs

They are more likely to have other medical problems which may be aggravated by antihypertensive therapy, eg, diabetes by diuretics or beta-blockers, or which involve the use of medications which may interfere with the therapy of hypertension, eg, NSAIDs with the action of diuretics, beta-blockers or ACE inhibitors.

Consideration of Drugs

The types of drugs used in the elderly need to be carefully considered. Doses of diuretics should be minimized so as not to decrease further a shrunken fluid volume but should be adequate to overcome reduced renal capacity to excrete sodium. Central agonists may further reduce mental alertness; beta-blockers may interfere with sleep and physical alertness. Initial experiences with calcium entry blockers have shown them to be particularly effective in the elderly. ACE inhibitors also work well; the compensatory shift in elimination provided by fosinopril makes it a logical choice in those with renal impairment.

Drugs should be given cautiously, with the initial goal of gradually and gently lowering SBP to below 160 mm Hg and DBP to below 95 mm Hg.

HYPERTENSION IN BLACKS

Blacks have more hypertension and suffer more hypertension-related morbidity and mortality than non-blacks. Both genetic and environmental factors are responsible for the higher incidence of hypertension, with high levels of stress related to minority status and poverty probably being involved. Restricted access to health care undoubtedly is involved in their higher mortality from hypertension since they are as well protected as are non-blacks when appropriate management is provided.

A stroke belt in the southeastern United States and a much higher prevalence of end-stage renal disease are two manifestations of the higher incidence of hypertension and the lesser access to therapy provided blacks in the United States.

Treatment should emphasize dietary sodium restriction since blacks tend to be more sodium sensitive. Their generally lower levels of plasma renin activity may reflect relative volume expansion and/or more extensive loss of renin-producing renal JG cells because of more extensive nephrosclerosis.

Blacks tend to be equally or more responsive to diuretics, alpha-blockers and calcium entry blockers but somewhat less responsive to beta-blockers and ACE inhibitors. This lesser responsiveness to drugs which act by suppressing the renin-angiotensin mechanism is in keeping with the lower PRA levels usually found in blacks. With a diuretic to stimulate PRA, they respond well to both beta-blockers and ACE inhibitors.

Of the secondary forms of hypertension, renovascular disease is less common, whereas renal parenchymal damage is more common. The latter may mainly reflect more hypertension-induced nephrosclerosis.

References

Aviv A, Aladjem M: Essential hypertension in blacks: Epidemiology, characteristics, and possible roles of racial differences in sodium, potassium, and calcium regulation. Cardiovasc Drugs Ther 1990;4(Suppl 2):335-342.

Finnegan TP, et al: Blood pressure measurement in the elderly: Correlation of arterial stiffness with difference between intra-arterial and cuff pressures. J Hypertension 1985;3:231-235.

Hofman A, et al: The natural history of blood pressure in childhood. Int J Epidemiol 1985;14:91-96.

Hulley SB, et al: Systolic Hypertension in the Elderly Program (SHEP): Antihypertensive efficacy of chlorthalidone. Am J Cardiol 1985;56:913-920.

Klag MJ, et al: The association of skin color with blood pressure in US blacks with low socioeconomic status. JAMA 1991;265:599-602.

Larochelle P, et al: Recommendations from the Consensus Conference on Hypertension in the Elderly. Can Med Assoc J 1986;135:741-745.

Messerli FH, Ventura HO, Amodeo C: Osler's maneuver and pseudohypertension. N Engl J Med 1985;312:1548-1551.

Plante GE, Dessurault DL: Hypertension in elderly patients: A comparative study between indapamide and hydrochlorothiazide. Am J Med 1988;84(Suppl 1B):98-103.

Rascher W, Gruskin AB: Recommendations for the treatment of hypertension in children and adolescents. Clin and Exper Hypertens 1986;A8:915-918.

Saunders E, et al: A comparison of the efficacy and safety of a beta-blocker, a calcium channel blocker, and a converting enzyme inhibitor in hypertensive blacks. Arch Intern Med 1990;150:1707-1713.

Tonino RP: Effect of physical training on the insulin resistance of aging. Am J Physiol 1989;256:E352-E356.

Tuck M, Janssens M: The differential efficacy of antihypertensive agents in the elderly. J Human Hypertens 1990;4:415-420.

#31 Special Patients: Diabetics

Clinical Information

Hypertension is more common among patients with diabetes and poses a major threat to the kidneys. The treatment of hypertension may aggravate glucose tolerance and interfere with the recovery from insulin-induced hypoglycemia. Obviously, diabetic hypertensives are a large and difficult group to manage.

Diabetes and Hypertension

Type I insulin-dependent diabetics do not have more hypertension until nephropathy begins, whereas Type II non-insulin dependent diabetics have more hypertension, probably because of concomitant obesity. The following increase the likelihood of hypertension:

- Older age
- Longer duration of diabetes
- Presence of proteinuria
- Obesity
- Female gender

Not only is hypertension more common among overt diabetics, but it is also more common among those with normal fasting blood sugars but with abnormal glucose tolerance tests. Such patients tend to be more obese. Obesity, hypertension and glucose intolerance may all reflect tissue insulin resistance.

Various diabetic complications may be accelerated by hypertension. The most striking acceleration has been in the progression of diabetic glomerulosclerosis, or Kimmelstiel-Wilson disease, which has become a major cause for end-stage renal disease (ESRD) as diabetics survive longer. Experimental data show that glomerularsclerosis is accelerated by hyperfusion of the capillary bed, as would be induced by high osmotic pressure from hyperglycemia and high intravascular pressure from hypertension. As will be noted, the progression of renal insufficiency has been slowed by effective antihypertensive therapy.

Antihypertensive Therapy for Diabetics

The blood pressure should be carefully controlled to prevent the progression of diabetic renal disease. Successful control of hypertension has been shown to slow the progressive fall in glomerular filtration rate and the amount of albuminuria in diabetics with nephropathy.

Problems with Drugs

Unfortunately, diabetics may be susceptible to various additional problems with many of the currently available antihypertensives. These problems include:

- Diuretics may worsen glucose tolerance and raise fasting blood sugars, probably by inducing hypokalemia which may further reduce insulin sensitivity
- Beta-blockers may blunt the effects of epinephrine needed to overcome insulin-induced hypoglycemia
- Both diuretics and beta-blockers may cause further derangements in blood lipids which are often abnormal in diabetics and further decrease insulin sensitivity
- Drugs such as central agonists and alpha-blockers may cause more postural hypertension
- High doses of ACE inhibitors may lead to more glomerular damage since they may cause a glomerulopathy, although this effect has not been shown to occur more frequently in diabetics given ACE inhibitors

On the other hand, ACE inhibitors have been found to reduce proteinuria and renal damage better than other antihypertensive drugs in hypertensive animals and to slow the loss of renal function in diabetic hypertensive patients. No hyperglycemic effect has been noted from the use of calcium entry blockers.

Therapy Guidelines

Non-insulin dependent diabetics may be safely treated with any antihypertensive agent but should be monitored for worsening of hyperglycemia and hyperlipidemia. Diuretic-induced hypokalemia should be prevented if possible and corrected if it occurs.

Insulin-dependent diabetics should be given beta-blockers with great caution.

All diabetics should be carefully checked for micro-albuminuria. If it is present, patients should be carefully controlled with the hope of preventing the progression of glomerulosclerosis. Studies are now underway to determine if special renal protection is provided by ACE inhibitors.

References

Bjorck S, et al: Contrasting effects of enalapril and metoprolol on proteinuria in diabetic nephropathy. Br Med J 1990; 300:904-907.

Christlieb AR: Treatment selection considerations for the hypertensive diabetic patient. Arch Intern Med 1990;150:1167-1174.

Dodson PM, Horton RC: The hypertension of diabetes mellitus: Mechanisms and implications. J Human Hypertens 1988; 1:241-247.

Klauser R, et al: Metabolic effects of isradipine versus hydrochlorothiazide in diabetes mellitus. Hypertension 1991;17:15-21.

Krolewski AS, et al: Predisposition to hypertension and susceptibility to renal disease in insulin-dependent diabetes mellitus. N Engl J Med 1988;318:140-145.

Luetscher JA, Kraemer FB: Microalbuminuria and increased plasma prorenin: Prevalence in diabetics followed up for four years. Arch Intern Med 1988;148:937-941.

Parving HH, et al: Effect of antihypertensive treatment on kidney function in diabetic nephropathy. Br Med J 1987; 294:1443-1447.

Tedde R, et al: Antihypertensive effect of insulin reduction in diabetic-hypertensive patients. Am J Hypertens 1989;2:163-170.

#32 Special Patients: Coronary Artery or Cerebral Vascular Disease

Clinical Information

Hypertension is the major risk factor for both coronary and cerebral vascular disease. Antihypertensive therapy will reduce the incidence of mortality from stroke. Protection from coronary disease by previously used therapies has not been conclusively demonstrated (see Section #11).

CORONARY ARTERY DISEASE

Clinical Information

Hypertensive patients with chronic stable angina should not be given direct vasodilators (hydralazine or minoxidil) unless the propensity of these drugs to stimulate sympathetic reflexes is covered by concomitant therapy with adrenergic inhibitors.

Hypertensive patients with atypical angina due to coronary spasm given beta-blockers may be susceptible to unopposed alpha-mediated vasoconstriction, although their reduction in myocardial work usually leads to reduction in anginal attacks.

Patients early in the course of an acute MI may have a marked hypertensive response from pain and stress-induced surges in catecholamine discharge. If the pressure remains very high despite relief of pain and anxiety, careful reduction of BP may be attempted under careful monitoring. Early use of beta-blockers has been advocated to reduce the extent of myocardial damage and may also be used to lower the BP. Unfortunately, the immediate antihypertensive effect of beta-blockers is usually minimal. Intravenous nitroglycerin or a calcium entry blocker may be better choices.

After the early period, continued use of oral beta-blockers has been shown to reduce recurrent MIs and mortality. Some patients who were hypertensive before an MI have a marked fall in BP post-MI, which may be a bad prognostic sign if it reflects impaired myocardial function. Use of ACE inhibitors post-MI has been shown to reduce the subsequent progression of myocardial dysfunction.

Reversal of Left Ventricular Hypertrophy

In addition to the use of beta-blockers and calcium entry blockers to reduce myocardial work and improve coronary blood flow in patients with coronary disease, various antihypertensive drugs have been shown to reverse the left ventricular hypertrophy (LVH) that is frequently noted by echocardiography, even in patients with relatively mild hypertension. Reversal has been seen with virtually all adrenergic inhibitors, ACE inhibitors and calcium entry blockers but not so uniformly with either diuretics or direct vasodilators.

Congestive Heart Failure

Various vasodilators have been found to reduce afterload and improve myocardial function in patients with congestive heart failure (CHF). The most impressive and sustained improvement has been noted with ACE inhibitors, and CHF is a major indication for the use of these agents.

CEREBRAL VASCULAR DISEASE

Clinical Information

Antihypertensive therapy has uniformly been found to reduce mortality from strokes. Despite occasional reports of overly-aggressive therapy producing either transient or permanent ischemic brain damage, the proper use of antihypertensive therapy is clearly indicated in patients with hypertension in association with TIAs or after a CVA.

32.

Acute Stroke

Caution is needed in the management of patients during the early course of a stroke. They may have transient rises in BP, presumably reflecting irritation of vasomotor centers or non-specific responses to stress.

Such rises may need to be gently lowered under careful monitoring, preferably with a parenteral agent, particularly if the patient is having intracranial hemorrhage. However, if the blood pressure is lowered and brain function deteriorates, the pressure should be allowed to rise to ensure that blood flow is not being further reduced.

Chronic Therapy

Cerebral blood flow (CBF) is kept very stable by adrenergically-regulated changes in the caliber of cerebral arteries and arterioles. The range of cerebral autoregulation in normotensive people is roughly between 70/40 and 180/110 mm Hg. Levels below the lower limits induce a fall in CBF with signs and symptoms of hypotension; levels above the upper limits induce hyperperfusion of the brain that is responsible for hypertensive encephalopathy (see Section #34).

Patients with chronic hypertension have a shift to the right of the entire curve, reflecting the structural thickening of cerebral arteries. The range wherein autoregulation maintains normal CBF may then be between 140/90 and 210/130. Sudden lowering of BP to below 140/90, though certainly not to a truly hypotensive level, may nonetheless induce cerebral hypoperfusion and bring on postural dizziness, weakness and faintness.

Fortunately, the range of cerebral autoregulation shifts back to the left with time, after persistent and gradual lowering of BP, presumably reflecting a decrease in the thickness of cerebral arteries. Thereby, lower levels of BP well into the truly normotensive range may then be tolerated. These findings may explain the frequent "washed-out" feelings that patients have when first using antihypertensive therapy that works too well. The better course is to go slow, bringing BP down only 5 to 10 mm Hg at a time, hopefully allowing CBF to be well maintained.

References

Anderson KM, et al: An updated coronary risk profile: A statement for health professionals. Circulation 1991;83:356-362

Barry DI: Cerebral blood flow in hypertension. J Cardiovasc Pharmacol 1985;7:S94-S98.

Bayliss J, et al: Clinical importance of the renin-angiotensin system in chronic heart failure: Double blind comparison of captopril and prazosin. Br Med J 1985;290:1861-1866.

Britton M, Carlsson A: Very high blood pressure in acute stroke. J Intern Med 1990;228:611-615.

Dunn FA, et al: Left ventricular hypertrophy and mortality in hypertension: An analysis of data from the Glasgow Blood Pressure Clinic. J Hypertens 1990;8:775-782.

Gillum RF: Stroke in blacks. Stroke 1988;19:1-9.

Kappelle LJ, et al: Transient ischaemic attacks and small-vessel disease. Lancet 1991;337:339-341.

Morgan HE, Baker KM: Cardiac hypertrophy. Mechanical, neural, and endocrine dependence. Circulation 1991;83:13-25.

Schlant RC: Reversal of left ventricular hypertrophy by drug treatment of hypertension. Chest 1985;88(Suppl):S194-S198.

Strandgaard S, Haunso: Why does antihypertensive treatment prevent stroke but not myocardial infarction. Lancet 1987; 2:658-660.

#33 Special Patients: Renal Insufficiency

Clinical Information

As noted in Section #5, progressive renal insufficiency is a common consequence of sustained hypertension, particularly in blacks who often have more nephrosclerosis than whites with similar degrees of hypertension. Half of blacks who reach end-stage renal disease (ESRD) that requires dialysis therapy do so as a result of hypertension. Although a smaller proportion of whites develop ESRD from their hypertension, this remains the most common preventable cause for ESRD.

The development of renal insufficiency tends to aggravate hypertension and may cause it de novo. Approximately 85 percent of patients with renal insufficiency will have hypertension, setting up the cycle of renal damage causing hypertension which causes renal damage. The process may involve sodium retention in most and the hypersecretion of renin in some. Patients with collagen vascular diseases may have rapidly accelerating hypertension because the intrarenal vascular disease activates renin release.

Control of Fluid Volume

Control of sodium intake and excretion becomes increasingly important as renal function worsens. Dietary sodium restriction should help, with the caution that overly rigorous restriction may cause those who have a fixed degree of sodium wastage to become volume depleted.

Diuretics are almost always needed. Thiazides generally work only if the glomerular filtration rate is above 30 mL/minute, reflected in a serum creatinine below 2.5 mg/dL. Those with more severe renal insufficiency will usually require a loop diuretic, although metolazone will work in many and requires only once-a-day dosage (see Section #14).

Other Therapy

In addition to adequate diuretic therapy, a number of other antihypertensive drugs may be tried, with no clear superiority of any other except for minoxidil. Most reserve this drug for those with severe hypertension, but it may prove useful in milder disease as well. ACE inhibitors may also be useful, particularly among those with a renin component to their hypertension. As noted in Section #23, renal function may suddenly worsen in patients given ACE inhibitors if previous high levels of angiotensin II were maintaining renal perfusion. This is most likely to occur in patients with bilateral renovascular disease or with a stenosis in the artery to a solitary kidney.

Overly aggressive falls in BP from any drug may, at least transiently, reduce renal blood flow and cause the serum creatinine to rise further. If the rise is not progressive or excessive, therapy should be continued since successful long-term control of hypertension may lead to an improvement of renal function. Such improvement has been noted less commonly than hoped for, perhaps because drugs have been used which further constrict renal vessels. Hopefully, the use of vasodilators such as ACE inhibitors or calcium blockers will provide better protection of renal function.

Doses of Drugs

Most antihypertensive drugs can be given in usual doses to patients with renal insufficiency. Exceptions include:

- Methyldopa
- Clonidine
- The water-soluble beta-blockers (atenolol and nadolol)
- Captopril

Doses of these drugs should be reduced by half or more in the presence of renal insufficiency.

33.

Dialysis and Transplantation

When renal function nears the end, dialysis is usually necessary to bring the blood pressure under control. In some, the response is dramatic. Hypertension that was unmanageable on three or four medications may become easily controlled on small doses of one or two. In others, however, the blood pressure remains a problem particularly on the days between dialyses. More careful dialysis by the chronic peritoneal route may provide better control of hypertension.

The implantation of a normal kidney may relieve or cure hypertension even if it began as the primary (idiopathic) form. This suggests that primary hypertension may start from renal dysfunction. Unfortunately, a number of events in the post-transplant period may bring hypertension back. These include:

- Cyclosporin therapy
- High doses of steroids
- Rejection
- Stenoses at the graft site

References

Bennett WM: Guide to drug dosage in renal failure. Clin Pharmacokinetics 1988;15:326-354.

Curtis JJ, et al: Hypertension after successful renal transplantation. Am J Med 1985;79:193-200.

Mourad G, Mimran A, Mion CM: Recovery of renal function in patients with accelerated malignant nephrosclerosis on maintenance dialysis with management of blood pressure by captopril. Nephron 1985;41:166-169.

Tolins JP, Raij L: Comparison of converting enzyme inhibitor and calcium channel blocker in hypertensive glomerular injury. Hypertension 1990;16:452-461.

Watnick TJ, et al: Microalbuminuria and hypertension in long-term renal donors. Transplantation 1988;45:59-65.

Zeller K, et al: Effect of restricting dietary protein on the progression of renal failure in patients with insulin-dependent diabetes mellitus. N Engl J Med 1991;324:78-84.

#34 Treatment of Hypertensive Crises

Emergencies vs. Urgencies

Some patients with markedly elevated blood pressures may pose a therapeutic emergency. Their blood pressures may need to be reduced within minutes if there is immediate danger to the brain, heart, or large vessel integrity or within hours if blood pressure is so high as to pose an eventual threat to vascular and target organ function. It is useful to segregate hypertensive "emergencies" from "urgencies" in selecting the best therapy:

- Hypertensive emergencies include:
  - Hypertensive encephalopathy, including eclampsia
  - Severe hypertension in the presence of active MI
  - Intracranial hemorrhage or dissecting aneurysms
  - Hypertension in the immediate postoperative period
- Hypertensive urgencies include:
  - Accelerated (Grade 3 fundi) or malignant (Grade 4) hypertension
  - Diastolic levels above 140 mm Hg
  - Congestive heart failure
  - Cerebral thrombosis
  - Rapidly advancing renal ischemia, eg, scleroderma crisis
  - Intractable nose bleed
  - MAO-tyramine interaction
  - Sympathomimetic drug overdose
  - Rebound from abrupt cessation of adrenergic inhibiting drugs

Drugs for Hypertensive Emergencies

When feasible, hypertensive emergency patients should:

- Be admitted to an intensive care unit
- Have an intra-arterial line inserted for constant monitoring of BP

- Be started on a parenteral agent (Table 34.1). In the past, this has usually been nitroprusside but labetalol or nicardipine may be equally as effective, easier to administer and safer

They should have the DBP lowered to a safe level (usually below 120 mm Hg) to remove the immediate danger but not so low as to reduce blood flow to vital organs. The safe diastolic level likely will be above 100 mm Hg.

If evidence of brain or heart ischemia develop, the pressure can be allowed to rise to see if the lower pressure is responsible. If not, the diastolic pressure should be kept between 100 and 110 mm Hg. Caution is needed not to reduce pressure too fast or too much.

Appropriate antihypertensive drugs should be started for more chronic therapy if the patient can take oral medication. IV furosemide may be needed to overcome the tendency toward fluid retention with successful lowering of the blood pressure. However, diuretics may not be indicated initially and may actually be contraindicated if the patient's fluid volume is depleted from prior GI or renal losses.

Drugs for Hypertensive Urgencies

Patients in less tenuous condition but with markedly high pressures have been successfully treated with numerous oral agents including:
- Clonidine
- Prazosin
- Captopril
- Minoxidil
- Nifedipine

Liquid nifedipine, extracted from the capsule and either placed under the tongue or swallowed, has been found to be particularly effective in rapidly bringing very high pressures down quickly and smoothly. Only 10 mg is usually needed, but that dose may be repeated in 30 minutes if an inadequate response to the initial dose is noted. Some, particularly if volume-depleted, will expe-

34.

rience too precipitous a fall with an initial 10 mg dose. An initial dose of 5 mg may be given. Captopril may also be used sublingually.

The goal of therapy is not simply to lower the high pressure but to institute an effective regimen for long-term control that the patient will take. This will require two or three oral drugs (see Sections #26 and #27). They can be started in small doses as soon as the pressure has been brought down from dangerously high levels and control has been achieved, verified by the patient's return one or two days after release from care.

As with all hypertensive patients, particularly with those who have lesser elevations, these patients should have the pressure brought down in a steady and gradual manner so as not to reduce cerebral and other organ blood flow too much, thereby making the patient dizzy, weak or sedated.

Evaluation for Causes

Patients seen for hypertensive crises must have careful examinations to uncover the underlying cause. Some may be obvious; however, renovascular disease is responsible in a significant number of patients, and a renal arteriogram should be done in all who do not have another obvious cause.

References

Ahmed MEK, et al: Lack of difference between malignant and accelerated hypertension. Br Med J 1986;292:235-237.

Bertel O, et al: Nifedipine in hypertensive emergencies. Br Med J 1983;286:19-21.

Calhoun DA, Oparil S: Treatment of hypertensive crisis. N Engl J Med 1990;323:1177-1183.

Chun G, Frishman WH: Rapid-acting parenteral antihypertensive agents. J Clin Pharmacol 1990;30:195-209.

Jarden JO, et al: Cerebrovascular aspects of converting-enzyme inhibition II: Blood-brain barrier permeability and effect of intracerebroventricular administration of captopril. J Hypertension 1984;2:599-604.

Kawazoe N, et al: Long-term prognosis of malignant hypertension: Difference between underlying diseases such as essential hypertension and chronic glomerulonephritis. Clin Nephrol 1988;29:53-57.

Lebel M, et al: Labetalol infusion in hypertensive emergencies. Clin Pharmacol Ther 1985;37:615-618.

TABLE 34.1 ➡

TABLE 34.1 – Drugs for Hypertensive Crises

Drug	Dosage	Onset of Action	Adverse Effects
Vasodilators			
Nitroprusside (Nipride, Nitropress)	0.5-10 microgram/kg/min as IV infusion	Instantaneous	Nausea, vomiting, muscle twitching, sweating, thiocyanate intoxication
Nitroglycerin	5-100 microgram/min as IV infusion	2-5 min	Bradycardia, tachycardia, flushing, headache, vomiting, methemoglobinemia
Hydralazine (Apresoline)	10-20 mg IV 10-50 mg IM	10 min 20-30 min	Tachycardia, flushing, headache, vomiting, aggravation of angina
Nicardipine	5-10 mg/hr IV	10 min	Tachycardia, headache, flushing, local phlebitis

166

Adrenergic Inhibitors

Phentolamine (Regitine)	5-15 mg IV	1-2 min	Tachycardia, flushing
Trimethaphan (Arfonad)	1-4 mg/min as IV infusion	5-10 min	Paresis of bowel and bladder, orthostatic hypotension, blurred vision, dry mouth
Labetalol (Normodyne, Trandate)	20-80 mg IV bolus every 10 minutes 2 mg/min IV infusion	5-10 min	Vomiting, scalp tingling, burning in throat and groin, postural hypotension, dizziness, nausea
Methyldopa (Aldomet)	250-500 mg IV infusion	2-3 hours	Drowsiness

ABBREVIATIONS

ACE	angiotensin-converting enzyme
ACTH	adrenocorticotropic hormone
BP	blood pressure
BUN	blood urea nitrogen
CBF	cerebral blood flow
CEB	calcium entry blockers
CHD	coronary heart disease
CHF	congestive heart failure
CNS	central nervous system
CT	computerized tomography
CVA	cerebrovascular accident
CVD	cardiovascular disease
DAVIT	The Danish Verapamil Infarction Trial
DBP	diastolic blood pressure
ESRD	end-stage renal disease
GFR	glomerular filtration rate
GI	gastrointestinal

(continued)

ABBREVIATIONS

HAPPHY Heart Attack Primary Prevention in Hypertension

HCT hydrochlorothiazide

HDFP Hypertension Detection and Followup Program

IPPPSH International Prospective Primary Prevention Study in Hypertension

ISA intrinsic sympathomimetic activity

IV intravenous

IVP intravenous pyelogram

JG juxtaglomerular

JNC Joint National Committee

KCl potassium chloride

LVH left ventricular hypertrophy

MAO monoamine oxidase

MAPHY Metoprolol Atherosclerosis Prevention in Hypertensives

MEA multiple endocrine adenoma

(continued)

ABBREVIATIONS

MI	myocardial infarction
MIBG	metaiodobenzyguanidine
MRC	Medical Research Council
MRFIT	Multiple Risk Factor Intervention Trial
NaCl	sodium chloride
NE	norepinephrine
NSAID	nonsteroidal anti-inflammatory drugs
PRA	plasma renin activity
RVH	renal vascular hypertension
SBP	systolic blood pressure
TIA	transient ischemic attack

NOTES

NOTES

NOTES

NOTES

NOTES

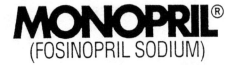

MONOPRIL®

(FOSINOPRIL SODIUM)

FULL PRESCRIBING
INFORMATION
ATTACHED